My Patients Like
TREATS

My Patients Like
TREATS

*Tales from a
House-Call Veterinarian*

Duncan MacVean, DVM

Skyhorse Publishing

Skyhorse Publishing books may be purchased in bulk at special discounts for sales promotion, corporate gifts, fund-raising, or educational purposes. Special editions can also be created to specifications. For details, contact the Special Sales Department, Skyhorse Publishing, 307 West 36th Street, 11th Floor, New York, NY 10018 or info@skyhorsepublishing.com.

Skyhorse® and Skyhorse Publishing® are registered trademarks of Skyhorse Publishing, Inc.®, a Delaware corporation.

Visit our website at www.skyhorsepublishing.com.

10 9 8 7 6 5 4 3 2 1

Library of Congress Cataloging-in-Publication Data

Names: MacVean, Duncan, author.
Title: My patients like treats: tales from a house-call veterinarian / Duncan MacVean, DVM.
Description: New York, New York: Skyhorse Publishing, Inc., [2018] | Identifiers: LCCN 2017054935 (print) | LCCN 2017058925 (ebook) | ISBN 9781510725683 (e-book) | ISBN 9781510725676 (hardcover: alk. paper) | ISBN 9781510725683 (ebook)
Subjects: LCSH: MacVean, Duncan. | Veterinarians—Biography.
Classification: LCC SF613.M28 (ebook) | LCC SF613.M28 A3 2018 (print) | DDC 636.089092 [B]—dc23
LC record available at https://lccn.loc.gov/2017054935

Cover design by Jane Sheppard
Cover photograph by iStock

Print ISBN: 978-1-5107-2567-6
eBook ISBN: 978-1-5107-2568-3

Printed in the United States of America.

Dedication

To Cruikshank and Charley, kindred spirits, like two peas in a pod.
Charley crossed the blessed Rainbow Bridge at 5:30 p.m. on November 3, 2012.
Cruickshank's story is yet to be told.

Contents

Preface

"What is your favorite experience?"—a question I am often asked and find difficult to answer. There are animals I've tangled with that I would just as soon forget, like the huge dog that mauled me over a mere vaccination. Of course, that was offset by a marvelous pig that listened to opera while I trimmed her nails. Most patients and their people are stories, wonderful stories, even when they are filled with pathos or turn out to be surprisingly bizarre. Like most of life's stories, truth is many times stranger than fiction.

My encounters have been rich, warm, humorous, and, at times, sad. It is these adventures, relationships actually, that I have endeavored to tell. The events are real, but names and certain identifying features have been changed so as not to compromise my clients' privacy. But those of you whom I've visited will, no doubt, recognize yourself and recall the events. A couple of chapters are comfortable amalgams of two patients and their people in order to more fully cover the issues involved and for educational purposes. In some situations, I disguised the breed or size of the pet, particularly where the telling may be embarrassing to my client and where nosy neighbors might otherwise figure it out. I retained the accuracy of the dialogue to the best of my ability. Any errors in recollection are mine alone. My remembrances may have been filtered by slight tweaking here and there; but the events, feelings, ambiance, and flavors are all there. Often the meaning of reality is brought into true focus through the lens of storytelling.

The general sense of how veterinarians do house calls and my own specific approaches are revealed through my stories. Additional details regarding the practice of veterinary medicine and house calls are included in the final chapter.

How did I begin? After leaving my professorship and academic life at Colorado State University in 1988, I moved back to my home-town of Sacramento, California. Wondering what to do with myself and wanting to refresh my clinical skills, I volunteered at various hospitals in the region. I am most grateful to all the local veteri-narians who let me observe, practice my skills, and probe them for knowledge.

I spent my first three years as a veterinarian working with wild-life in the jungles of Malaysia. My pre-veterinary undergraduate degree was in wildlife conservation, with hands-on capturing and handling many exotic species. One of the doctors who helped me with getting back into clinical medicine and surgery suggested that I start a house-call practice. He pointed out that I could start with minimal financial investment and that my wildlife veterinary expe-rience would be useful in dealing with exotic species and fractious pets. I've never regretted this career change, which has provided exciting challenges and variety and has been so rewarding in the people and pets I've met.

I've been treating and handing out treats to animals in my house-call practice for over twenty-five years now. These creatures in our care are wondrous. And so are their human companions. Our pets protect us, they work for us, they play with us, and they perform for us. And just as importantly, and in many cases *more* importantly, they aid our health, both mental and physical. Companions—that is what I endeavor to tell about in this book.

As companions, these furred, feathered, and scaled species are indeed full members of our families. I've always had difficulty calling us "owners." Owners we are not, any more than we are owners of an adopted child. No, we are responsible for them. We are caretakers.

Who are the caretakers I've encountered in my practice? There is no specific classification I can give them. Most are animal lovers, but not all. True caretakers do love their pets. Most have real empathy for their pets, but not all. Some clients are caretakers by default, such as when parents "inherit" a ten-year-old pet parrot (which might live for another thirty to forty years!) when their child leaves for college. One client received custody, when her ex-husband died, of a twenty-year-old green-winged macaw that could live for another fifty to eighty years—and the parrot didn't like her.

Many people assume that the majority of house-call clients are shut-ins or elderly. That was not the case with my clientele.

My most common clients, no matter what part of town they lived in, were busy working people with several pets, who preferred the efficiency and convenience of having a house call as opposed to hauling the brood, one by one, to a veterinary hospital. They found that, with so many animals averaging out the added fee of a home visit, the cost wasn't much different from what a hospital would charge for the same services and meds.

A common visit for me consisted of annual checkups for dogs and cats, which included physical examinations and routine vaccinations. It often went like this—

Pushing my way through the front door so the dog(s) or cat wouldn't run outside. Dogs and a curious cat sniffing my pant legs and my medical satchel. Some dogs scratching at my bag to get at the treats sequestered there. Skittish cats scurrying away to another room or under some piece of furniture. Questions from kids wanting to listen to heart-beats through my stethoscope. Holding, or restraining, often struggling, to keep a wiggly dog or nervous cat in place so I could inject the vaccines. Often having my client help, and sometimes having to teach how to hold, which might require fetching a dog's collar or scruff a cat's loose skin between the shoulder blades. I can't count the number of times I had to explain how scruffing does not hurt the cat and how natu-ral it is since it is the way momma cats move their kittens around. Doing the exams in a well-lit area (a challenge in homes where the lighting is poor; sometimes I did this out in the backyard if there was still daylight or by flashlight if it was dark). Many times conducting the exams while I knelt or lay down at pet level. Frequently, I got the "While you're here, Doc, could you also take a look at Peaches? She's not due for shots, but she's been scratching at her ears a lot lately." All of these could happen in a single day's visits.

Those types of visits were the more typical. And they could be ex-citing, even before ringing the doorbell, anticipating what lurked behind the door. Many times the experiences might start out in a typical fashion and then turn out to be a comedy or tragedy or just plain creepy. In the following chapters, I open the door for you to peek in on my world as a traveling vet.

I
Dogs and Cats Reign

"A dog iz the only animal kritter, who luvs yu more than he luvs himself."

—Josh Billings

"Thousands of years ago, cats were worshiped as gods. Cats have never forgotten this."

—Terry Pratchett

1

The Dog with No Teeth

One boiling summer day, I was driving to Rio Linda, a small town northwest of Sacramento, on an emergency call to see a dog that was reportedly hemorrhaging from the neck and rump.

The heat was rising in waves, with houses at the distant end of the road forming shimmering double images reflecting off melting pavement. It is easy to get around town as the streets are sequentially numbered and laid out in a more or less rectangular grid. However, finding a particular address can be a challenge. Many of the houses don't have numbers on their mailboxes, on the street, or on the houses. Some don't have mailboxes, and many houses are set back a ways from the road.

Rio Linda became populated in the 1930s by immigrants from midwestern and southern Dust Bowl states. Advertisements promised rich California farmland. The migrants arrived only to find that the soil was a mere two- to six-inch veneer over impenetrable hardpan, in which only weeds and a rare stunted tree could survive. Even so, these rugged latter-day pioneers erected homes and raised families, forming a colony that some called poor white trash—but actually was a proud, tenacious people struggling to provide for themselves and their families. They built their small, handcrafted homes out of what was available and put down their roots in the hardpan.

Land and housing in the area are still among the least expensive in the state, partly because of the soil, frequent flooding due to overflowing creeks, and lack of a significant tax base. Some homes are upscale; most are not. Many of the residents are would-be farmers with small acreage, housing livestock, horses, chickens, and the usual cats and dogs.

I slowed down as I came to each house that didn't have an easily visible address. My sudden slowing to a crawl as I strained to make out a faded mailbox number upset a fellow in a pickup behind me. The driver honked, but as I didn't speed up, he took out his irritation at this slowpoke by honking and spinning wheels past me, giving me the ol' finger, and yelling some profanity I didn't care to make out.

Just as I was getting a headache trying to figure out the numbers, I found the place, sitting between houses reading 1640 and 1680. *Yep, 1660 it must be.*

I pulled into the dirt driveway, up to a gray prime-patched Mustang on blocks and an engine hanging on a hook from a pulley in front of a doorless garage. Some chickens scratched in the driveway, clucking in satisfaction at pecking a bug or piece of corn while others squawked out back of the garage. The air was scented with a confusing mixture of sweet bird feed and sour grease. All manner of car carcasses were corralled inside the corrugated metal walls of the garage, an obvious add-on to the '30s vintage wood-frame house. A workbench lined the wood wall that was the north end of the house. Handy, well-used workman's tools were scattered over the dark, oily surface of the bench.

To my right, the front yard was surrounded by a five-foot-high chain-link fence. Some grass, mostly bare dirt. A stunted Sacramento cottonwood tree stood on the street side of the yard. It was the only shade. The cottonwood was shedding, providing white flocks of floating floss to form snowy drifts along the fence and to land like dander on all that came near.

I braced as I stepped out of the comfort of my air-conditioned car into the oven outdoors. Zipping up my smock and grabbing my medical bag out of the backseat, I stepped around the Mustang and turned toward the gate. Caution had taught me to approach slowly and wait until I was sure the way was not guarded by a "nice" dog. Sometimes I've entered a yard where the caretaker has assured me how nice the dog is that I was coming to see, only to be greeted by a snarling, slobbering mass of canine muscle looking more like a creature out of a movie like *Alien*. Other times, it has been the "other" dog, the one not mentioned but sharing the same premises.

Out of the front door of the slatted-frame house ran a barefoot woman in a blue and white tank top and a thin pink skirt that tightly snugged her trim body. As she quickly approached, I noticed emblazoned across her bosom an emblem denoting the event of the year in Rio Linda—the Little League parade, picnic, and festivities heralding the initiation of the season of team play.

She was in her twenties or early thirties, tall, maybe five-ten, waving her arms above her head, shaking.

"Oh, Doc, ah'm so glad y'all's heah at last. My dawg is bleedin' somthin' terr'ble."

"It's all right, Mrs. Dennis, we'll see if we can just fix him up fine." Inhaling deeply, trying to find something personal to comment on to make connection, "By the way, I like your accent. Where are you from?"

She seemed to settle at this. She shook my hand while opening the creaking gate that could have used a little WD-40. Her pretty face visibly relaxed, dark brown eyes dancing, a wide smile lit up between her high cheekbones like a sun breaking through a storm cloud. "Well, thank ye. Ah'm from Tenn'ssee, up in the Noaweast hilly paht."

The line of her lips hardly concealed a straight row of teeth with a few gaps that winded an occasional whistle between certain words. She started telling me her account, assisted by Italian-like hand animation. Her Alaskan malamute, Randy, was in the front yard that morning when she came outside to throw some corn in the driveway for the chickens. "He's jus' sittin' thar, blood all ov'r his nick, and sittin' in his haunches in blood. I grab 'is collar and yanked 'im insahde t' th' kitchin, 'n washed his nick and rear end. He still got blood on' im, Doc. Ya gotta do somthin'."

The wooden boards of the stairs to the front porch were loose, some warped, and a few boards were missing. The white paint was faded and cracked; the curtain in the porch window to the right of the screen door was fluttering out through a break in the glass. A standing fan was whirring like a propeller beyond the curtain. Beside the fan was a couch that was sagging with age and comfort in what looked like a living room area. Through the torn screen door that was flaked with fluffy white cotton, I could see a straight hallway down to what looked like another screen door at the back of the house. Light shined on the dark wood floor. Framed pictures hung straight and orderly on dark walls.

"Bring Randy out here on the lawn where it is well lit. I should be able to see his wounds real good out here."

She ducked inside for a few seconds and then appeared on the porch, bent over, holding the malamute by his collar. She dragged him across the porch like a mop, down the stairs, and onto the grassy part of the yard. "Now y'all sit 'n mind th' doc. He's heah t' help ya."

With that, she let go, and the dog just sat there, long, thick, sleek gray coat and panting with tongue drooping out. Clean teeth, two or three years old, ears erect, steel eyes attentive.

I looked Randy over and palpated his body, feeling for swellings and wet spots. There were two streaks of blood staining the fur about halfway up the front of his neck. I couldn't detect anything out of place or abnormal on any other part of the body. Lifting him up from his sitting position, I saw a smudge of red on his rump but didn't detect any wounds there. I peeked under his belly and tail. Intact male. No injuries underneath.

"Mrs. Dennis, I'm going to get my electric razor out of the car to shave his neck and take a look at the wounds. All I've found so far is blood on his neck. Maybe the smear of blood on his rump is just blood that fell to the ground that he sat on. Do you have an electric outlet nearby that I can plug into? And can you get me a pan or bucket of tap water?"

"M'be ya kin use the lahght cord from the grahj my hubby uses t' work on his cahrs." Then she ducked inside the house for the water.

I retrieved the electric razor from my materials-and-supplies box in the trunk. I took the extension cord leading up to the frame of the Mustang, plugged it in, and took it through the gate as far as the cord let me.

She came out shortly with steaming water. I told her, "Good. Set th' bucket over thar next t' the fence." I blushed. Dern, I was beginning to sound like her. My internal dialogue flurried through my skull. *No, not mocking,* my mind defends, *just connecting with her through identifying language, you know. Oh, crap,* rebuts my heart, *you just blurted it out. Be yourself, man. All right, I got caught up in the middle of the colorful language of the moment.* Not so bad.

I watched my tongue and said, "Bring Randy over, so I can shave him."

She dragged him as before over to the edge of the lawn near the gate. It took a while to shave through the thick coat enough to get to the skin and see the extent of the wounds.

I thought to myself how, if I were Randy, I'd want to be indoors by the fan, not out here in the valley heat. Whew—in my smock that felt by then as thick as a malamute's coat, I was dripping sweat and beginning to pant myself. The cottonwood shade fell just short of us.

There were two fresh puncture wounds at mid-ventral neck, one on each side of the trachea. They were oozing a little blood, but not bad. They had missed the jugulars. One of the holes was a jagged laceration and might require one or two sutures. I thought they should heal all right after washing, disinfecting, and giving an antibiotic injection. "Ma'am, these are punctures, and . . ."

She caught her breath, inhaling while blurting out, "How could thar be punctuals? They look like holes. How'd that happen? Who did that?"

"No, ma'am," I interrupted, "they are holes. Probably bite wounds. The holes are from being punctured by teeth about as far apart as a good-sized dog. Not deep enough as a cat or raccoon. Probably a dog."

"But, that cain't be. They's no othah dawg could git in ta th' yahrd. I make good sure o' that one."

Earlier, through the screen into the backyard, I had seen what I thought was a dog. I asked, "Do you have another dog?"

"Well, yes, but he couldna done it." Shaking her head, knowing where my question was leading.

"Is it the dog I saw in the backyard? It looked like a pit bull."

"He is. Do y'wanna see 'im? He's a love, as gentle as kin be. Bull and Randy play all th' time."

She disappeared into the house while I went back to the car for some scrub disinfectant, syringes of local anesthetic and antibiotic, and a laceration repair kit.

I arrived back at Randy just as the Mrs. appeared back in the yard, leading a squat, muscle-solid Bull. Bull's wide body approached, wagging his surprisingly thin tail and slobbering the back of my outstretched hand. Yep, a pit bull—and intact. "Do they play roughhouse sometimes?"

"Oh, yes, theys acts as if thar goin t' tar each other apart. Theys roll 'round on the ground shakin' each othah."

"My guess is that Bull bit Randy while playing rough."

"No, sir, ain't no way he coulda dun it." Her jaw now set defensively.

Raising my eyebrows, I said, "But look, he is strong, low to the ground, and could easily grab Randy at throat level and break the skin, even with a playful bite. He has strong jaw muscles."

"But, Doc, he's over fahve yar old. He goin' on eight. He coulna done it. No way, no how."

"Why would five years make any difference? He is still strong, and he looks healthy to me."

"Yep, he's healthy. I raised 'im m'self! B'fore we moved heah from Campt'n two yars ago." As if that answered my question. She stood there, hands on hips. "Are ya goin' stitch 'im up?"

I knelt down, turned to Randy, and started scrubbing his neck with disinfectant. "But I still want to know why Bull could not have bitten Randy."

With a look at me as if I was dumber than a nail, she answered, "'Cuz he ain't got no teef!"

"What do you mean, no teeth?"

Still looking at me as a nail, she replied, "No dawg in Campt'n has any teef aftah theyen fahve yars old."

Stubbornly, "And why would five years make any difference?"

"Ev'r'one knows they chews on rocks 'n gravel 'n' they ain't no more teef left by time they git t' fahve."

Well, I thought, the proof is in the pudding they say, or in the mouth in this case. I stood up and walked over to Bull, gave him a reassuring pat, really reassuring myself his disposition was all right. He looked relaxed and friendly enough. I bent over, pushing down on his lower jaw with my left hand and, with the fingers of my right hand, pushing the edges of the lips inward between my fingers and the crown of the teeth behind the canines. I pressed my fingertips upward on the roof of the mouth to stimulate the jaw opening reflex. With figurative fingers in my mind crossed, I said, "Say ahhh!"

Whew: Bull opened wide in a brilliant yawn. Pit bulls in my experience often are stubborn and lock their jaws, and I can't get my fingers inside the mouth enough to evoke the reflex.

As if looking a gift horse in the mouth, I peered in. Tilting my head aside and splaying the gaping mouth in full view, I announced with victorious flair as if amplified through a bullhorn, "It looks like a mighty fine set of teeth to me, Mrs. Dennis."

With consternation awash all over her face as she looked on, she said, "Well, I'll be goldern. He's got teef."

"Yeah, his teeth are worn down a little but still sharp enough to break skin with the strength of a pit bull's jaw. His upper canines are just about as far apart as the two punctures on Randy's neck."

"Yar mahghty rahght, Doc, theyr's teef." Pausing, relaxing her jaw, "I guess he coulda done it aft'r all." Turning to Bull, "Ya caint play rough like that no more, y' heah?"

The lady then expressed concern that sometimes Bull gets out of the yard and might cause trouble down the neighborhood, now that he has teeth that is. Her thought was how he could have hurt that sweet chow bitch that he was hooked to when she was in heat last year.

I continued, "And are lots of the dogs in Camden also coprophagous?"

"Cop o' what?"

"Do they sometimes eat their own or other dog's crap?"

"Yep, theya showly do. I doan wanna go looking in theyar mouths!"

I was smiling inside, thinking about what it must be like in the part of the world she grew up in, with dogs running around with dentures ground down to the gums. Lots of young dogs chew on rocks, especially if bored. But in some of the hill areas in the

Appalachians, the soil is mineral-deficient, I recalled reading some-where. And in some of those remote areas, people feed pets what-ever scraps there are, and the pets just have to do with whatever they can find. It seemed to me that eating, or at least chewing on, rocks and feces seems like a useful way of attempting to supplement the diet, for those dogs anyway.

I proceeded with injecting the local anesthetic and the antibi-otic. While the painkiller was taking effect, I told her how the dogs' being males and still having testicles could contribute to their ag-gressiveness. I urged her to consider getting both dogs neutered. "Once they are fixed, they may be calmer and less likely to inflict serious injury to each other. And they might be more inclined to stick around the house and not wander off when the air fills with a whiff of a bitch in heat or where they could trouble other dogs or people in the neighborhood." I didn't bother to add that it also would eliminate the possibility of testicular cancer.

She stared, narrowing her eyelids. "Ya mean gittin' them casted?"

"Uh, castrated. Yes, surgically removing their testicles. It doesn't hurt them since they are under full anesthesia, and recovery is quite smooth."

"Oh, no, my husband says he's not gonna let anyone do that to 'em."

"Why not?" knowing full well the likely answer.

"He says, 'No one's gonna cut my balls out an' they ain't gonna do it t' m' dawgs neithah.'"

I laughed. That's a common identification men make with their pets. I didn't respond, knowing I would be wasting my time trying to reverse those hormone-driven convictions.

I went ahead and trimmed the jagged edge of the laceration on Randy and placed a single skin suture. I showed that wonderfully worthy woman how, in ten days, to get scissors and cut the stitch on one side of the knot and, holding the knot, to pull the suture straight up, away from the skin, to remove it. That way, I wouldn't have to make another house call simply to remove the suture.

She disappeared into the house to get cash to pay me while I finished cleaning up and hauled my bag and instruments back to the car.

We were saying our good-byes when her husband arrived, pulling up beside my car. He drove an old blue Ford pickup with dents and scratches, a workingman's truck. He revved the engine before killing the ignition. Almost jumping out of the truck, he came over to the gate, holding out his hand. I shook his strong grip. His calloused fingers that had hard-earned grime under the nails wrapped around my hand. There was a deer-like creature tattooed on his forearm. He had a one-day growth of dark beard, stood about two inches shorter than his wife, and wore a faded green T-shirt with the name of some band I'd not heard of with pictures of a banjo player and fiddler around the name. His pants were soiled blue jeans, his shoes scuffed black. His smile was as wide as his wife's, sans two upper middle incisors. "Hi, m' name's Jimbo. Ah see you stitched up m' dawg," glancing over to the shaved neck.

"Pleased to meet you, sir. It looks like you've been working hard on your car?" I said, nodding toward the Mustang. He smiled with pride, rubbing his hands together. He and his wife seemed to be good, hardworking people, doing the best they could, with love for their animals. Love for each other was confirmed by the obvious affectionate look he gave his wife as he turned and headed for the garage.

I thanked the wife as she thanked me. I felt good. Nice people.

Feeling a breeze that had just come up, it didn't seem so hot anymore.

I drove out onto the pavement, stirring up dust as I left the driveway. I pondered and smiled at the lesson I'd learned today about the dogs with no teeth, and the dirt, stools, and rocks they chewed on.

2

Pussycat, Pussycat

Where have you been?

David and Sarah Robinson, expatriates from Berkeley, California, were friends of ours. They lived at the top of the hill only a few houses from us in Petaling Jaya, Malaysia. Though they were fifteen years senior to us, my wife and I were invited from time to time to social activities at their home. Their functions were mostly cocktail parties at which CEOs, lawyers, doctors, politicians, ambassadors, and other VIPs were the attendees. My wife, Anne, and I suspected we were included in the entourage not simply because we were neighbors. They knew that my wife's father had been chief justice in Singapore, an island nation located at the tip of the Malay Peninsula, in the years immediately prior to the Japanese invasion in World War II.

I was their veterinarian, seeing their cat, Pussycat, from time to time for routine house calls, occasionally treating her for chronic gingivitis, a common problem in the breed. She was a gorgeous Abyssinian with gold-brown fur and a white blaze at the base of her neck. Her eyes were a stunningly bright green. She was independent as hell and did not like me handling her on my vet visits.

The Robinsons catered to influential people with style at their home, which some guests called "The Mansion." Among those entertained at their home were US colonels and generals who had come down on brief furloughs from the Vietnam War to Kuala Lumpur for rest and recreation. David and Sarah were vibrant and lavish hosts.

I was in Malaysia, working as a staff veterinarian on a tropical medical research project. It was my first job after graduation from veterinary medical school. I was striving to further hone my clinical skills by working on the side. To do that, I volunteered to work with the veterinarian at the National Zoo and took house calls for the pets of fellow employees on the medical research project I worked on. I also attended to the pets of American embassy personnel and others, like the Robinsons, who asked for my services.

Mr. Robinson literally fit the "tall, dark, and handsome" modicum. He was a "businessman," as he put it, who did business with the US government and various foreign entities. This required that he travel a lot. One day, as we made small talk, sipping our pink gins (straight gin with a drop of grenadine) at one of his Sunday afternoon curry parties, he confided to me that he even "slipped" into some geographic localities where Americans are persona non grata. It never was clear to me exactly what business he was in. "I connect business with business," is how he put it to me. He had a firm handshake, a smooth tongue and wit, and a smile to make you feel comfortably welcome at his home.

Mrs. Robinson was, as she put it, "just along for the ride." She said they had moved around a lot and lived in countries too numerous to count. She was expected to host parties for "dignitaries and other important people," she said. It seemed to me she was the ultimate partner for the handsome businessman—always the lithe model, dressed in the latest fashions, with an outgoing and warm personality to make anyone feel special at whatever event she hosted. She was tall, slim, and beautiful, with an eye for beauty in her surroundings so that the Mansion was a furnishings and artistic showcase.

On this New Year's night, it was hot. The air was laden with intense humidity after a brief but violent storm we had that afternoon. Lightning forked and crackled across the sky. As is common in the tropics, the heavens emptied buckets of water.

I was sleeping restlessly, tossing and turning in my sweat. The phone on the bedside stand rang. I reached under the mosquito netting and grabbed it after one ring, not wanting to wake my wife, who was sleeping in the other twin bed. I glanced at the alarm clock next to the phone. My eyes read a blurry 1:00 a.m.

It was Sarah. She needed me to come over for an emergency concerning her cat. I could not ignore her call for help as she sounded desperate and said it was "urgent." Even if it was the middle of the night. *Oh well, I'm not sleeping anyway.*

Lifting the mosquito netting and trying not to wake my wife, I slowly eased off my squeaky mattress. I slipped on a light pair of khaki shorts, not bothering with underwear, *just another layer*, and a colorful short-sleeved cotton shirt (*can't go to Mrs. Robinson's house wearing a plain shirt*), stuck my feet into the rubber flip-flops at the foot of the bed, stood, and rubbed my eyes awake. I walked downstairs in the dimness, not bothering to switch on any lights, grabbed my satchel and my small insulated box in which I kept my most commonly used pharmaceuticals and instruments, and headed out the door. I didn't know what to expect as Sarah was so brief over the phone.

Damn, I'm barely awake and it's dark out here. This had better be good, I thought, as I stumbled out of the house to the car, lugging the two bags.

Then the better part of my brain kicked in. I chastised myself for even thinking of the bother of a nighttime call ahead of my patient's and my friend's concerns. *Emergencies*, I tried to tell myself, *are just part of the job. I like being of service. And it's only a short distance up the road.*

I started to perk up and didn't miss the sweaty bed and mosquito netting anyway. It was dark as a cave as there were no streetlamps in this suburb of Kuala Lumpur. My headlights shined like beams through the air—air so humid it was more like a steamy fog. The street surface glistened from remnants of the storm.

After parking in the driveway that curved in front of the Robinsons' estate, I saw that the porch lights were out. No light shone from the living room window. I thought of how Dave must have had trouble, because of the storm, getting his flight out for one of his many business trips. *Maybe the electricity was out and wasn't repaired yet.*

I rang the doorbell, medical bag in hand, leaving the pharmacy in my car. No answer. It was then I noticed the door was ajar. *Not good.* Puss-Puss (a name I'd heard the Robinsons call their cat) could escape to the grounds, and she was strictly an indoor cat.

Sarah's voice called from inside, "Come on in, Duncan, and close the door." Her voice like a trace of incense in the air came from upstairs. "Come up here. In our room."

I had visited the house often enough that I knew the master bedroom was the third door on the left at the top of the stairs. I walked over the travertine tiles past the marbled pillars of the entryway. The hallway leading to the stairway was decorated with original paintings, hung in pleasing spacing, like a museum.

The curved tile staircase was well lit with candles emitting the smell of vanilla and a hint of rose. Flickering pairs were placed every few steps, and there were several on small shelves along the wall leading up the stairs.

As I made my way, holding onto the dark walnut banister, I mused, *What a wonderful soft glow and feeling candles give, and the dizzying aromas . . .*

"Hurry in here!"

My reverie startled, I thought practically. *Of course, we keep candles for emergencies like storm blackouts.* I quickly made my way along the corridor, which was lit with candles like an airport runway to the open bedroom door. The interior of the room had a few candles lit, but fewer than along the previous path so that I could barely see in the dimness. Sarah was limned in the soft glow as she sat at the foot of the bed. I could make out that she was wearing a silver satin nightgown that shimmered in the dancing candlelight. She patted the bed beside her.

I glanced around the room for her cat.

"The bed, Duncan," Sarah said softly.

A lot of my feline patients that are sick or scared scoot under beds. I set my satchel down and took out a penlight.

I got down on my knees, lifted the bed skirt, and took a peek underneath. I called out, "Here, Puss-Puss; here, Puss-Puss." *I know cats don't come when called unless I rattle a food bowl, but, oh, well.* Of course, no response.

No cat at the end of the bed, no cat at the head, and no telltale lump suspending down from the mattress lining (a favorite hiding spot of some pets).

From underneath, I called up to Sarah. "I can't find Pussycat anywhere under here. Did you see her go underneath?" No response. "Maybe she's gone into hiding in the closet?"

"No, here," she answered. Her voice had the quiet tone of her normal sultry lilt, but with a hint of the raspiness of exasperation.

Then, as I was bringing my head out from under the bed, I heard a faint squeak of what I thought was a bedspring. I looked under again. Nothing. *Maybe she came out of hiding and had jumped onto the bed. Great.* Abyssinians are fond of crawling under covers. I smiled. I pulled my head out from underneath, stood up, and looked.

There was Sarah, sprawled on the bed with the sheets pulled back. The flimsy thin nightgown that clung to her shapely body had the bottom edge rumpled up to her waist. Sarah squirmed her hips in a sexy shift and spread her thighs wide apart. Her arms reached up toward me. She smiled, her lips curled, and she mewed, "Meow."

My jaw fell open. I was dumbfounded. I started to say something. My throat choking, I just stuttered, "Sssarrahhh . . ."

Even in the dim candlelight I could see her smile, with tongue licking her lower lip, and gesture with her finger as she said in as breathy of a voice as I've ever heard, "Come, here, my young man, my pussy needs you. Feed me."

My head was swimming, I felt faint witnessing the sultry surprise lying there lifting her butt ever so slightly off the sheet toward me. I didn't know what to say. Sure, I had admired her good looks and enjoyed her mild feminine flirting before, but I'd never looked at Sarah in a sensual way.

But, I did feel heat rising in my groin. *No, this can't be.* The tropical heat was not enough to melt the shock that froze my tongue. My mind froze as well, but thankfully, my body didn't.

Some propriety in me flooded the muscles of my legs; I grabbed my bag and backed out of the room. I hurried down the candlelit stairs and out into the dark where my lungs desperately sucked in the thick humid air as if I had not inhaled since my insipid cry of her name.

I climbed into the car and started the engine. My body was trembling. Nothing like that had happened to me. Never before had I been approached so blatantly. Although married, I still felt somewhat naïve back then in terms of male-female nuances of interaction. Especially the idea of an older married woman with a young married man. On the way home, my face flushed, sweat oozed out of my skin. I felt so embarrassed.

When I arrived home and walked into our bedroom, my heart pounding like a freight train, my wife called out from underneath the sheets, "How did it go with Pussycat tonight?"

I flushed again and looked the other way, hurrying to the bathroom. "Okay. Nothing wrong. I took care of it."

But I didn't. I was sure even in the darkness she could see the flush in my face. I stayed in the bathroom quite a while. Until she fell into slumber. Then I crawled into bed for a fitful sleep.

A few weeks later, my wife informed me that she accepted an invitation to a party at the Robinsons', the usual cocktail party with some of their "connected" friends. The latter seemed to be important to my wife. I tried thinking of some excuse not to go but couldn't manage it. *How would I face Dave—let alone Sarah?*

As it turned out, Sarah acted as if nothing happened. Her greeting was the usual one when we were received at her parties, especially when guests were within earshot, "Good evening, *Dr.* and Mrs. MacVean." Her hug was no friendlier than usual, accompanied with the gratuitous kiss in the air with cheeks barely touching. Dave's hand reached out in a welcoming grasp, warm and firm. He seemed none the wiser. *Whew!*

Events at which we would see the two of them became less and less frequent while more and more Chinese and Vietnamese guests revolved in and out of their house over the ensuing months. Dave spent more time away than at home. Within a year, the Robinsons moved.

Without leaving a forwarding address. And Pussycat went with them.

3

Them

"Hello, this is Dr. MacVean. How may I help you?"

"Can you come over? Something's happened to my dog Shadow."

"Have I seen Shadow before?"

"Well, yeah. Doc, Something bad has"—phone static sounds—"Shadow. Come over now."

"Let's start with you tell me your name. Then tell me what you need."

"It's me, Billy. You know, from Arbor Lane."

"Oh." The street name rang a bell. *That Billy*, I thought. His mom, Arlene, was the one who always phoned before. "Okay, Billy. What's up?"

"He's . . ." More static.

"I didn't catch that. Phone static."

"Yeah, it's the interference. I said, 'He's been killed.'"

"I'm sorry, Billy, so sorry," feeling hit in the gut. *Such a magnificent dog.* "What can I do for you?"

"Is he dead? He's been killed. How'd they do it? Why? You can do an autopsy."

"Well, I could come over now, and we'll see what needs to be done. Give me about half an hour."

"Okay. But hurry."

I gathered my medical satchel and tucked it into the trunk of my car. The drive was quiet through streets at dusk, the time of no shadows. My drive was only three miles to Del Paso Heights, a business and residential district north of Sacramento. As I drove in, it appeared somewhat blighted but with hope from the new tenants, artists and poets taking up residence and putting galleries together.

When I was a boy growing up in the city, this area—"The Heights" as my parents called it—housed a racetrack and a bowling alley. As I bumped over the tracks that once had been streetcar steel, memories rose of the smell of exhaust fumes from midget autos spinning around the track, kicking up clouds of dust, and of the crack of pins flying as my mom's sharp curveball smacked the pins during moonlight bowling night.

Pulling myself back from memories, I wondered what Billy really wanted. Usually his mother would phone, as she seemed to take responsibility for their two dogs' feeding, grooming, and treatment. Billy just sort of lived in his mother's house. No job, no apparent duties other than maintaining the yard once in a while.

I pulled up to the chain-link fence surrounding the house and parked on the gravel depression that marked the entrance that once was a driveway. No car was parked on the grounds now.

Grabbing my grip, I approached the gate. The weeds were overgrown, sticking through the links like discarded straws. The unkempt yard was six to eight inches high with foxtail grasses and star thistle. A narrow path worn down to dirt led from the gate to the side of the faded yellow wood-frame house. The path now bypassed the front porch it led to three years ago when I was last here to give rabies shots. I unhooked the gate latch, pushing wildness aside to pass, and squeezed my way through.

The porch railing needs fixing. The house and grounds have deteriorated since I was last here. What's going on?

I walked to the back of the house where the path turned left to the back door. Another path led from the door to the field that was once a backyard. I knocked.

Billy opened the door, very slowly, only an inch or two, and looked out to see who was there, his eyes flittering back and forth. He reached out with his short muscular arms and waved his fat fingers, motioning me into the house.

"Hi, Billy, how are you?"

He said nothing, just opened the door. He peered around me as if checking to see if anyone else was behind me. Satisfied that I came alone, looking right and left, up and down; he stepped aside to let me pass. He left the door wide open and brushed past me.

Billy Blake was a stocky young man of thirty years or so, with a short-sloped forehead, chubby cheeks, and broad nose. His long blond hair was tied into a ponytail that curved limply over his left shoulder. Below thick eyebrows, his eyes were dark as coal and reflected the world as if shielding his soul. When he spoke, his round head bobbled and appeared to be doing a balancing act on top of a broad stalk of a neck. He was barrel-chested with a beer belly. Thick legs supported his five-and-a-half-foot frame. I expected to see him barefooted, wearing a white T-shirt and short Levi cutoffs—his usual attire.

In a hoarse whisper, glancing back out the door, he said, "I need to see who's coming."

Puzzled, I asked, "Who are you expecting? Is your mom . . .?"

"No, no, she's gone." *Well, maybe that explains the lack of yard maintenance.*

Billy looked different from how I'd seen him before. There were furrows in his brow. He wore a long-sleeved white shirt, stiff-starched but wrinkled, as if he'd been sleeping in it. Sleeves buttoned. A loosened bow tie hung around his neck. Long black pants with cuffs. Black, he'd revealed to me once, was his favorite color. Black shoes, but stark white socks. A black suit coat hung on a chair in a corner. He looked like he'd been to a funeral.

Furtively glancing around the kitchen/dining area where we stood, he pointed to the middle of the room and said, "There. Is he dead? Look him over good, Doc. I know they did something to him."

The room was dark, except for the TV off to my right, emitting static from the snowy screen. I told him to turn on the light so I could examine the body. The room smelled of unwashed clothes and mildew.

Shadow, a huge, intact, male, twelve-year-old German shepherd, lay on his left side. Stiff, legs straight out as if in spasm. Rigor mortis. Acrid smell. Tongue flopped out of the right side of his mouth. *Curious.* It's as if the tongue was pulled out and placed on the right since he was lying on his left side. The jaw was set but not clenched shut. No apparent discharge from eyes, ears, mouth, or rear quarters. No apparent injury to skin. I took out my stethoscope and knelt down beside the large form. As I placed the bell of the scope onto his chest, I could feel he was icy. There was no more heartbeat than I expected.

"I knew they did it."

What's he talking about? "Did you move him? Or did he die here?"

"Right there . . . I think. He might have been moved by them."

"What do you mean?"

Glancing all around the room, lowering his whisper even further, "It was them. I know it. They did it."

"Who? Who are you talking about?" A little loud and exasperated.

"Shh. Don't let them hear you. They don't know I called. I went to a pay phone because mine is tapped. They know everything. But not everything. They don't know you are here."

A clipped silence and a glance out the back door. "What did they do to my dog?" He fidgeted with the collar of his stiff shirt. He stared down at poor stiff Shadow. *Dead over an hour ago.*

A magnificently proud dog, Shadow. He carried tall, straight back, only slight curve of rump to rear legs. Well-muscled. Ears erect, attentive. Deep chest, straight front limbs. Strong muzzle and gleaming white teeth set in firm jaws. Show-dog qualities. All of this apparent now, even in the distance of death.

"Billy, Shadow is dead. I'm not finding anything specific to point to cause of death. I'll turn him over. Maybe there are clues, Billy."

"BILL. It's BILL!" he said, jumping up and down and waving his arms about wildly. "I'm Bill. I'm not Mommy's little boy. Not anymore!"

"Okay, okay," I said with as calm a voice as I could muster. *Just a minute ago and on the phone, you were Billy.* I bent down and slowly turned Shadow over, keeping an eye on poor Billy.

Billy backed away, edging toward the wall near the door to a small spare room. The dining area was converted into a sort of sitting room: a couch against the wall near the back door, the kitchen to the right. Opposite the couch was a wide archway into what once was a living room. That entry was mostly blocked by a bunk bed, like two banks of teeth opening into the maw.

On my previous visits, Arlene Blake usually sat with legs dangling over the edge of the top bunk. She said she slept there, and her son slept on the bottom bunk. She was thin with a gray complexion, looking much older than her fifty or so years. The beds were always in a state of dishevelment, unmade. A stuffed toy shepherd dog was always somewhere near the pillow at the head of the lower bunk.

The TV, which was turned off on prior visits, sat in an alcove to the right of the beds, partially in the kitchen. There was a door in the wall to the left. They said it was a storage closet. The door was always closed. A rectangular rug lay in front of the couch. No coffee table. A yellow Formica dinette set was stuffed into the small kitchen area to the right of the back door. I had always before entered the house through the front door, passed through the living room that was piled with a jumble of old papers, magazines, blankets, chairs, and table, and then walked along a path through the mingle-mangle and past the end of the bunk bed into the dining area.

Sparky, their other pet, an overstuffed American Eskimo dog, used to run up to greet me and jump up to lick my face as I bent down to pet him.

"By the way, where is Sparky?"

"Oh, he died. I buried him in the backyard." His hand waved toward the open door.

I looked back out the door. Two mounds, packed dirt. Beside them was fresh earth, piled high beside a large hole in the ground. I guessed for burying Shadow.

"I took Shadow earlier today to the police station. I asked them to protect him from them. They just laughed and tied my hair up into this frizzy ponytail."

"Who did?"

"The police."

What? Strange man. I shrugged my shoulders and got on with my job.

I lifted the stiff post-like front legs and easily rolled the big guy over onto his right side. Examination results were the same on this side. Nothing.

"Bill," I emphasized with a louder tone than usual, "Shadow may well have died suddenly, but I'm not finding anything specific."

"But they killed him, and they tortured him. They rammed iron rods down his throat until he gagged. Then they shoved an ice pick up his rear end. Blood was gushing out, and Shadow was howling. Then the noise stopped." Billy's head drooped, his eyes closed, his arms shaking.

I didn't see any blood on the floor. I took out my penlight and peered into Shadow's mouth—all intact with no evidence of trauma. I looked over his rectum. No trauma. I donned a latex glove, lubed a finger with K-Y jelly, and digitally explored his rectum—no palpable tear or irregularity and no smear of blood on the glove when I pulled out. "There is no evidence he died the way you say he did, Bill." I offered to perform a necropsy, cutting the carcass open to determine pathogenic or traumatic lesions.

"But I know they did it. They hid a microphone in his collar, and when I would walk him, they would tell me things through the collar." He glanced around the room. "I told the police, but they wouldn't listen." His eyelids tightened to angry slits.

He sat down on the couch, fidgeted, and silently motioned me over to him. I hesitated, just for a moment, and then sat beside him, with worry crossing my mind. He began to elaborate, whispering and glancing around the room the whole time.

"They must have killed him. They've been out to get me."

Must be some kind of harmless paranoia, I reasoned. I relaxed. No edge.

He pointed to the corners of the ceiling. "Up there, they have microphones, with silver wires that cross the attic. And there are magnetic plates under the floorboards. They hear me. They're listening right now." His eyes grew big as saucers as he turned to look at the television of snow pattern and static. He clenched his fists.

My neck muscles tightened. The hair began to stand up on the back of my neck. I felt the chill of fear.

"Do you hear that?"

"What?"

"They're talking to me out of the TV. *EEEeeeehh*. Stop it. Stop it," clasping his hands over his ears.

I stood up. The fear in his face mirrored the fear inside me. I squirmed.

"Now, Bill. Take it easy. Just relax. It will be all right." *Convincing myself?* "It's okay. Your mom will be home soon. It'll be okay," I said, trying in vain to stay calm and relaxed.

He moved his hands to his lap. His face flattened. I inched slowly toward the back door. It was dark outside now. He continued in a low whisper, very calm.

"No, Mommy's not coming home. She went away. She's gone."

Suddenly it dawned on me. My heart skipped a beat as I glanced out to the darkness through the back door. *Two* mounds. And a fresh grave yawning its black gape for another body.

My voice quavered, "Where is your mom? Where has she gone?"

He answered in a low monotone, looking down at the floor, unsmiling, a dead look in his eyes. "Mommy's gone now. Gone."

Gooseflesh covered my arms, back, and legs, and dread chilled my spine. Mouth going dry, trying not to let my fear show. My voice cracked, "Well, I don't think I can help you. I'd best be going now to my next appointment." There was no appointment, but I wanted to get the hell out of there. I bent over to zip my bag and pick it up, keeping a wide eye on Billy. *Forget my fee. I'm out of here.*

As I backed toward the door, I calculated I had a second or two before he could spring up from the couch. *If I can just keep a few steps ahead of him . . .*

"Wait! I have the money. Just wait right there, and I'll get it." He jumped up from the couch, arms waving, eyes wide, looking sideways at the TV. Some distant voice in his ear.

Startled, I cried, "No, it's okay, Bill. Pay me later." *But I'm never coming back here again.*

"No. No. I have it. Right here in the closet." He motioned toward the storage room door.

Good. I'll have even more distance from him as I make my escape.

He smiled, whispering, "Yes, yes," and backed away, opening the storage door, his eyes on me.

Good God. A gun? A knife? Keep going, back into that room. That's it. A little farther.

I was unexpectedly glued in place, breathless, an anaconda wrapped around my arms and chest. Couldn't move. Joints locked. I felt like a captive waiting for execution. Wide-eyed, I stared as one hand reached into the top drawer that he quickly pulled open with his other hand. The object he drew out was dark, long, and pointed. A strange thought came to my mind of a mini samurai.

"No, no. I'll send you the bill." Now my legs loosened and stretched into backward strides, toward the back door.

Then, I saw that what he held in his hand was a scroll. He turned it on edge, and out plopped a bundle of bills. He threw the scroll onto the couch in a jerky motion. At that, I almost jumped. He then started peeling off dollar bills. "What do I owe you?"

Seeing he had nothing else in his hand, I answered, "Eighty will do." *What are you doing? Just get the hell out of here.*

He whispered, quite calmly now. "Do you know how the Mafia makes money? They tip the police as to what's goin' down. They send radio waves through the aquifer. You just need to send an antenna down to the water table, and you can listen to what they say."

What the . . . ? This guy is certifiably nuts.

He opened the bundle all the way and lifted the inside bill out, handing me a C-note. Still coming toward me. "Keep the change."

I never grabbed a fee and headed out so fast in my life. I was practically running out the door. I rounded the corner at a jogging pace, down the side of the house, stumbling in the dark. My toe caught in a tangle of weeds, and I tried shaking loose while looking back to see if he was following. I pulled my shoe free, turning to look back at where I'd come from one more time before sprinting to my car. I spun and took off, looking over my shoulder. Then, *wham!* I bumped into something solid—in the middle of the path.

There stood Billy, standing firm, legs straddling the line to the car. His hands on hips, glaring.

"God, Billy"—*oops*—"what are you doing? You scared the skin off me!" I looked him over to see what he had in his hands. In the dark, I couldn't be sure what he had. He must have come out the front. We were opposite the porch, and I could see the door was ajar.

Billy leaned toward me, moving hands to thighs, a kind of linebacker stance. He panted, "You forgot to say good-bye." He extended one hand toward me in a handshake position.

"What?"

"It's okay now. They can't hear us. The wires are all inside, and I'm not wearing the hat that tells me things. I left it on the couch. It gives me awful headaches." He shook his head side to side. "I want to thank you for showing me how they killed my dogs."

I shook his hand lightly, with just the fingertips, while pulling my bag up, waist high between him and me. *Showed you how. . .? Just get me out of here.* Gathering all the strength and matter-of-factness my voice could muster: "You're welcome. Gotta get going."

"Bye-bye." He stepped to one side, toward the house, wiping his brow with one hand and pointing at the sky with the other. At God only knows what. Whispering.

I edged my way around him, still keeping my grip between us, looking back and forth from Billy to the gate, a mere ten yards away. So as not to put my back to him again, I walked sideways to my car, my head swiveling back and forth as if at a tennis match.

When I finished latching the gate, I looked back. He was gazing upward, swinging his arms in an arc, whispering something.

I couldn't resist. "Bye, Bill. Who are you talking to?"

"THEM."

4

Mr. Grey

Mr. Grey was referred to me by the Northgate Pet Hospital that was just three blocks away from where Mrs. Simmons lived. Her Mr. Grey, a dull charcoal-colored, long-haired cat with enormous yellow eyes, was in so much pain she was afraid to pick him up to bring him in to her regular veterinarian. As the Mrs. said when she called me, "Mr. Grey yowls real loud when I pet him. I can't cuddle him anymore, and he won't let me brush him."

I arrived, medical bag in hand, with syringes, needles, and blood and tissue collection vials, fully expecting to take samples for laboratory testing. Even before meeting Mr. Grey, I introduced myself and asked the usual questions regarding age and gender. Then came the questions of history, such as origin and prior medical problems.

She was anxious and got immediately down to describing her cat's current condition. Responding to my questioning, she replied, "Yes, he's restless. He won't stay in one spot very long, and he's really fidgety. He runs and hides from me. But there are other times he just acts lazy."

Mr. Grey sauntered out from the kitchen with head held high as if he was in charge of who came and went in this house. He brushed by, tentatively rubbing against my pants leg, sniffing the smells of other patients who'd done the same thing earlier in the day.

Mrs. Simmons, a spry seventy-year-old whose gray hair was fastened into a bun, was tall but thin as a wisp. She became upset when Mr. Grey cried out in pain when I picked him up. I placed him onto the kitchen countertop for the examination. As I ran my hand over his body, I noticed his haircoat was dull, and he had flaky dandruff. His ears felt hot to me. *Likely a fever.*

In a loud voice belying her slender and delicate-looking stature, she told me to stop "poking" him. A reasonable request from her point of view. *But it's my job.*

When I probed about diet, she told me he had stopped eating. With a sad look on her face, she shook her head side to side and added, "And I feed him only his favorite. Tuna. I give him the best canned tuna money can buy. Human grade, not just that tuna-flavored cat food. He's always liked tuna before. What cat doesn't like tuna?"

"Well, actually, not all cats like tuna. Some don't even like any kind of fish."

"Yes, finicky cats. But not my Mr. He's sick," she said, nodding. Her head wobbled on her pencil-thin neck and looked like it might topple off.

I released my grasp on Mr. Grey's scruff when I reached for my satchel to get out my stethoscope and otoscope. Mr. Grey yelped as he squirmed loose, jumped off the table, and scurried off down the hall.

After several minutes of searching each room that had an open door to the long hallway, we found him in the back room hiding under a bed that was nestled up against the corner of the room. We both crouched on our hands and knees, head down and butts in the air like a pair of feeding ducks, peering into the dark chasm under the bed. Yellow eyes stared back at us.

I thought of how I wouldn't be able to bribe him to come out from his secure cave with food. *She said he wasn't eating.* I started talking to myself about whether or not I would need a broom to flush him out so I could finish the exam. *I can't go around to his side without moving the bed away from the wall.*

She heard my mumbling and wagged her finger at me. "No, you don't. Don't you dare hurt him again," in an admonishing tone as if I was a cruel animal abuser.

"It's okay. At least," I told her, "I know what is likely wrong with him."

She said, quite firmly, "Then you really don't need to examine him any further."

Mustering up my best "Doctor" look, I told her the reason I would still like to examine him is that I wanted to be sure nothing else was bothering him.

"Oh, it might be something other than what you think is 'likely' causing the pain?" emphasizing the word likely.

I reassured her, "I'm pretty confident as to what the problem is, but I need to finish the exam." We got off our knees and sat on the floor on the rug beside the bed.

"Can you cure it?"

"Yes, I think so." Not as unsure of myself as that answer sounded. She caught it, that little nuance of phrasing that we use to hedge our bets.

As I was gathering my thoughts, pondering what way to best express my conviction, she interjected, "Well, what's wrong?"

"Tuna," I responded. "It's the tuna."

"What? Poisoned tuna? It's a can from Safeway." She paused, adjusted her sitting position on the floor. Then, placing her hands on her hips and squinting at me, she said, "Really, Doctor, how can it be poison?"

Good question. "It's not poison. The tuna is not poisoned. It's just that if a cat eats tuna almost exclusively, over time its metabolism changes in a way that causes inflammation of the body fat. Mr.

Grey has this condition, steatitis, also called yellow fat disease. He's in pain because his body fat is inflamed. Kinda like his fat tissue is burning up inside."

She was upset at the idea of her cat burning inside. But, at the same time, she was fascinated that a fish, which she believed all cats love, could make him sick.

I added, "Even cats without much body fat, like Mr. Grey, can suffer from this. Not all cats love fish, even tuna. But don't you just love cats—so independent, so different? Lovely personalities." And, before I let her jump in and enumerate the exceptions, I assured her Mr. Grey would return to his old self if she would eliminate tuna from his diet. "Tuna is deficient in vitamin E, and the high unsaturated fats in tuna deplete the vitamin E even more. Steatitis can result in death if left untreated."

A worried look flooded her face. "He won't eat anything else. You know how finicky cats can be about their food, and Mr. Grey really *loves* tuna."

"And cats can become addicted to tuna—a 'tuna junkie,' as it were."

I gave her some suggestions of what to buy at the store to feed Mr. Grey, letting her know that most modern commercial cat foods contain enough vitamin E. Tuna-flavored cat food is not 100 percent tuna and has other meats and nutrients that are necessary in the feline diet. I added that other, non-oily fish with low unsaturated fat don't cause steatitis. I told her to get some vitamin E, 200 International Units per capsule. Then, twice during the next week, cut the end off a capsule, squeeze a drop or two of the oil onto Mr. Grey's food, and mix it in. "It will speed up Mr. Grey's recovery."

We were still sitting on the floor, nodding our heads, beginning to come to some consensus. I then gave her my view that animals get bored with the same food over and over. "We don't like eating the same thing, meal after meal. Variety is good. You can feed fish, as an occasional treat, but do it in moderation."

"Yes, I know that one," she smiled. And with a twinkle in her eye, she explained, "My mother used to say it when she drank her sherry at night before bed—'Sin, but in moderation.'"

We both laughed. *We're on track together.* I decided to let well enough alone and not pick up Mr. Grey to finish the exam.

She was delighted that there was a cure for him and that Mr. Grey would bounce back to his old cuddly but feisty self.

We got up off the rug, went into the kitchen, sat down at her dinette, and talked for a while. I told her how yellow fat disease was common a couple of decades ago but not anymore. Human-grade tuna is fed much less often as the sole diet nowadays.

We reminisced how tuna was cheap back when we were kids but no longer. You could get different grades of tuna, five cans for a dollar. Cans of tuna are now smaller and more expensive. I remembered, when I was a kid, how often my family had an inexpensive meal of creamed tuna on toast for dinner. Now it's pricey.

Mrs. Simmons pushed her chair back, stood up, and asked if I was hungry. "It's lunchtime."

I was, I told her.

She said, "Good. I'll fix lunch."

"I don't have much time," I said. "I'm running a little late on my appointments." *As usual.*

She reassured me. "Oh, it won't take time at all. It's just a sandwich, and you can take it with you."

"Okay, that would be great."

"TUNA sandwich! And I already have a can open," her mouth expanded into as wide a grin as I've ever seen.

I can hardly believe how much I belly-laughed over that one.

It was a good sandwich, the way I like it—lots of relish, mayo, mustard, and a crunchy touch of chopped celery.

5

He's Never Done That Before

When I arrived at the sprawling white stucco house after a long winding drive through the countryside, Ms. Lyle was waiting at her front doorway. I got out of my truck, picked up my clipboard with attached patient form and medical bag, and walked up the step-stone path. She appeared to be in her sixties, short peppered hair, barely five feet tall. Her slim frame looked frail, with narrow shoulders. Bending over a chow with golden-fleeced mane, she told him I was a friend and "He's here to visit us. Be nice; he is okay."

She tugged at his leash and led him over to me. I stopped and let him sniff my pants legs, so he could read the smells of other dogs I'd seen that morning. He sniffed the back of my hand, which I extended very cautiously. *She had to tell him to "be nice"?*

She told me his story. At least, what she knew of it.

Mr. Chow, whom her neighbors just called "Dog," was abandoned by a family who moved away over a year ago. Ms. L. and other neighbors fed Mr. Chow but couldn't catch him to take him in. Ms. L. was finally able to coax him into her yard by dropping a trail of food bits. She quickly shut the gate behind her. Eventually she was able to pet him and brush him, "somewhat" as she put it.

Her smile faded when she told me that she was worried because his coat was shedding in clumps, and there seemed to be a different-colored layer underneath. She wondered if he was sick. In her sugary, high-pitched voice she told me he has been the "sweetest, nicest dog."

After we got inside the house and found a well-lit place to do the physical examination, I approached him. He snarled and growled. I backed off. Ms. L. said, "He's never done that before."

I raised my eyebrows. *How often have I heard that? Only countless times.*

Like a pebble dropped into a pool of still water, remembrance rippled to the worst bite I ever received. I was sent back to the time when a diminutive Asian woman introduced me to her "sweet, loving" Akita in her backyard on a thick-coat December day. Blackjack, whom she called her lucky dog, was an unneutered male with a black-and-white haircoat. He was massive, over 150 pounds. He didn't look at me and just paced back and forth. The small lady stood next to him (like David next to Goliath) as I had asked her to. I told her to try to keep him in one spot, so I could give him the needed rabies vaccination.

I was loading the syringe and didn't see her pick up a bone from the porch railing. Just as I leaned forward toward the dog and pinched the skin to insert the needle, she threw the bone down at his feet (to distract him from the needle prick, she later told me). Thinking I was going after his bone, the dog suddenly turned on me, rearing up to full height, and charged, pounding his front paws into my chest, nearly knocking me over, and pushing his head forward with jaws wide open, lunging toward my throat.

I instinctively raised my arm to protect myself; his teeth clamped down, biting through my jacket and into my forearm. He kept chewing, shredding through the padded nylon of my jacket, ferociously trying to get at my face and throat. I backed up as fast as I could toward the side door to the garage. The dog kept pushing forward with his hind legs, paws on my chest, mouth on my arm, the two of us in a macabre dance.

My back slammed into the door; I frantically twisted the knob with my free hand. As the door gave way, I backed in, pushing his bulk away from me as best I could. Finally, I was able to close the door between my arm and his head. As he fell back from the door, jaw clenched, my jacket sleeve went with him.

It was then, as I stood there shaking, that I saw the blood run down over my hand and onto the floor. I had not felt any pain in the adrenaline rush to protect myself. But then, seeing the wetness drip onto the floor, throbbing pain splashed into my consciousness.

I whipped off my jacket and rushed into the kitchen to wash my wounds in the sink. I stared down at the rivulets of red clouding the cold water. I barely comprehended the sight, with torn edges of nerve and tendons twitching like worms in the holes in my flesh.

I shook myself out of the shock, picked up my bag, and drove myself to the hospital. It took several sutures to close the gaping bite wounds. When I took my shirt off in the ER, I saw there were indentations of paws three inches wide on my chest, with toes and nails clearly visible. For weeks, I carried bruises on my chest as if a dog dipped his paws in ink to leave his signature.

Shaking off the thoughts of punctures past, I said, "I think we'd best muzzle Mr. Chow before I examine him. And I think he will need a sedative injection."

Ms. L. looked distressed. "Oh, poor thing. To have to have a muzzle. Are you sure? He'll be all right. I gave him a tranquilizer pill an hour ago to calm him down."

Calm him down? From what? She knew.

"I'll be right back. I'll just get the muzzle from the truck and then show you how to put it on." As soon as I said that, a worried look washed over her face. Did it come from fear, I wondered, or did she feel bad that Mr. Chow would suffer the indignity of having to wear a muzzle, or something else? Maybe she sensed my apprehension. I certainly had reason to distrust dogs with bushy up-curled tails, like chows (and Akitas). My duty (I was clear on that) was to make sure that neither I nor Ms. L. got bitten by a pet that had "never done that before."

When I returned, I had her put a leash on him. I then took the leash from her and showed her how to put the muzzle on. I assured her he would not be able to bite once the muzzle was secure. *Now, if she can just get it on properly without spooking Mr. Chow. We might not get a second chance.*

She hesitated, seemingly fearful of her own dog. She reached into a pocket and produced a Milk-Bone treat, which the dog snapped up. I was nervous, remembering that bone-Akita action. But she managed to slip the plastic cage of the muzzle over Mr. Chow's nose and jaw and started to buckle the strap. I pushed the strap down below the ears, as she had it over the flap of the ears where it might easily slip off, and buckled it up tight—not an easy thing to do without ensnarling the long fine fur of a chow in the buckle and strap.

We were ready. I drew up a dose of sedative into a syringe and approached Mr. Chow's hindquarters. She held the leash, up near the neck like I showed her, so he would have less space to move in. He was okay . . . until the needle touched his skin. Then he jumped, swinging his rear away from me and turning his head to face me. Ms. L. held the leash tight.

Mr. Chow and I did a little dance for a while, back and forth, with me chasing his rump, until I finally got the injection into a back muscle. We led him out onto the patio where there was good lighting and removed the muzzle. Since the drug would take at least ten minutes to take effect, we started to fill out the paperwork—outside, where I could keep an eye on Mr.

When she asked how long the rabies vaccine would be good for, I realized I'd forgotten my vaccines when I left the house. *Oh, no, I'm a good twenty minutes away, each direction. I'll just have to suck it up and go get them.* That morning, when I was preparing to leave for my house calls, my mind was elsewhere. I was thinking of some bills that needed paying rather than paying attention to gathering all the supplies I needed for the day. *Now all my other appointments will be backed up. It will be a long day.*

I excused myself, explaining in my apology to Ms. L. that I forgot the vaccines. She very kindly empathized and, with a wink, assured me with tongue-in-cheek that "In all my years, I've never known anyone else that forgot something on the way out of the house!"

Musing that vote of confidence, I left. *I'm sure he'll be knocked out from the sedative until I get back. Not to worry. Cross my fingers.*

Of course, as things always seem to go when you're in a hurry, I slogged along to my home office behind slowpokes and logging trucks. On the way back, taking a road I believed would be a short-cut, I got stuck waiting in a line behind a road repair crew. My angst stirred again. *The sedative might wear off, and Mr. Chow probably would not let me get the muzzle on a second time.*

I tried to console myself by thinking about how every animal's individual response to drugs was different—what's called idiosyncrasy. Maybe the tranquilizer my client gave him would prolong the action of my sedative. Or maybe the time it would take for the drug to take initial effect would prolong the total time. I bet on the idiosyncrasy. I hoped.

I arrived on the back patio with the vaccines. Mr. Chow was snoozing away, lying on his belly, snoring with his head resting on his front legs. Ms. L. told me, "He just went to sleep a few minutes ago. It sure took a long time for him to get drunk and then pass out."

Good, maybe we'll have enough time to get the exam and vaccinations done.

I suggested putting a blanket or towel over his head, just in case. "It always seems to quiet a pet down."

"No, I'm sure that won't be necessary. He's out cold."

Hmmm, I wondered.

With stethoscope in hand, I listened to his chest. Slow, but not too slow, steady, and strong heartbeat. Lung sounds were soft and normal. Then, in a test of the depth of his sedation, I lifted him somewhat as I pushed my hands along both sides of his flanks and felt his abdomen. Pulling up on the belly enough to feel internal organs, carefully, slowly, not to arouse him. *Good, no obvious masses or abnormalities. Now the touchy part.* Lifting his tail. No visible lesions. *Skip the rectal palpation. No use taking a chance on waking him with* that *intrusion.* The fur was coming off and exposed the thick undercoat of a chow.

"Don't worry about the shedding, ma'am. The coat looks healthy underneath. A normal darker color. Summer shedding."

"Oh, thank you. I was so worried about it. What about his mouth? Shall I help open his jaws?"

God, no! "Wel-l-l, we will just lift up his head, and I'll take a peek at his gums and teeth." I reached for a tongue depressor. *It would be good to lift his lips for a quick look.*

As I kneeled down in front of him, Ms. L. reached down and put a hand under his chin and lifted it. Then, as quick as a rattlesnake strike, he snapped at her, just missing her hand. And before I could stop her, she reached again for his chin. This time, he nailed her. The arch of his teeth tattooed red spots on her hand. She gasped, then leaped away, tripping over Mr. Chow's head, and lunged forward, crashing to the brick pavement, hitting her head on the leg of a nearby table, and falling on her left shoulder.

It seemed like it took a couple of seconds for me to realize that she was down. My mouth gaped. Shaking my head out of the shock, I jumped up and went to lift her slight body off the pavement, away from Mr. Chow. But she rolled over and waved me off, saying, "Don't touch me. I'm okay." *Strange. But some people are touchy. How bad is she hurt?*

All I could manage to blurt out was, "Are you sure? Are you sure you're okay?" I felt confused at her not wanting my help. Of course she was in shock, but it might be a concussion, I thought.

No redness or cuts appeared on her forehead where she hit the table.

I grabbed a blanket from the couch just inside the sliding glass door and threw it over the dog's head. *I can't take care of her, but I can take care that Mr. Chow doesn't attempt to bite. Covering his head so it's dark will calm him back to sleep.* I hoped.

She closed her eyes, lying on her back. She put her right arm over her face, shielding her eyes. "Don't try to move me. Please. I just need to lie here a moment. I think my arm is broken."

Helpless, I stood there. With a possibly fractured arm, moving could be painful, I rationalized. I glanced back and saw that the form under the blanket was not moving.

"Are you sure? I could help you sit up. Then when you're ready, I could help you stand," I persisted, offering my arm down to her.

"No, no. I just need to rest. My left arm hurts. I can't move it."

"No, I would take you by your right side and lift you gently. I . . ."

Interrupting, managing a smile, she said, "What about 'No' do you not understand?"

I couldn't stifle a laugh. I relaxed and stepped back, throwing in a little humor of my own. "Well, at least I got a glimpse of his teeth. Hardly any tartar!"

But at the same time, I felt bad. *How much do I force, or do I simply leave her alone?* I wondered how stubborn she could be. Of course, she thought I was stubborn to persist against her "No." I had to say something helpful. "We've got to get your bite wound washed. Thoroughly, with soap and water."

Moan. "Yes, okay. In a minute." Turning a suspicious eye toward me, thinking I might try to lift her, she continued, "I'll get up on my own."

I was concerned she would lose her balance again. *What the heck, I might as well get on with the vaccination.* There didn't seem to be anything I could do for her. It appeared she was just going to continue lying there.

I went ahead and gave the distemper and rabies inoculations. As I was filling out the rabies certificate, which she would need to license the dog, Ms. L. sat up. Once more waving off my gesture to help, she pulled herself up with her right arm on the table. She stood steady. "Would you please get me an ice pack? There's a towel in the drawer to the left of the sink and an ice dispenser in the fridge door."

I asked, "Can you raise your left elbow sideways? Maybe it's a torn rotator cuff rather than a fracture."

She couldn't. "Dr. MacVean, either way, it hurts, and I won't be using my arm for a while. The ice pack?"

I insisted on washing her hand. She relented and walked with me to the sink. There were no tears, just small shallow indentations. *Sutures would not be needed.*

I applied the ice pack to her shoulder, and she held it there with her good hand. "That feels better," she sighed.

As she sat down in an easy chair in the living room, she went on to tell me that she was current on tetanus shots. She'd just gotten one last spring.

I had to ask, "Why did you need a tetanus shot?"

"Poor Mr. Chow nipped at me. I was taking up his food bowl to wash it, and he jumped up and caught my elbow. But it hardly broke the skin and healed up real fast."

"So this was not your first encounter with Mr. Chow's teeth." But, "*He's never done that before*"?

A kettle of water was sitting on her stove. "I see some tea on the shelf. I'll fix you a cup."

I was about to turn on the burner when she stopped me, saying, "No, don't. I don't want a cup of tea now."

"It's the Brits' cure for everything."

"Well, I'm not English, maybe a little *Scot*-tainted, Dr. *Mac*, but I don't care for anything. You help yourself to whatever you want."

I got a glass of water and joined her in the living room. She went on to tell me more. "Last month, my grandchildren were visiting. Mr. Chow rushed at my grandson. I had to step between them to keep him from being bitten. In June, my gardener, who was helping me rake up lawn clippings, was attacked—a real nasty bite, on the leg."

That was enough. Feeling anger rise, I said, "Maybe you should consider putting him to sleep. Your grandkids are not safe around him." *That's an understatement! And why did you put on the charade that he'd never bitten anyone?* I presumed she was in doubt about whether or not I would let him be my patient if I knew he was aggressive.

"Oh, I know. My neighbors tell me I should. I've noticed him getting more and more aggressive since he's been here. I love him so. But maybe I should. Not let him wake up. I know. I'm told a lawsuit is around the corner if he keeps . . . My gardener was real nice. He just let me pay for his doctoring up."

"I have to phone my clients for today and tell them I'll be considerably delayed or reschedule their appointments." Still feeling responsible, I added, "I want to drive you to your doctor or an emergency room."

"No, I have a friend down the street who drives me to my doctor. He will take me." Shaking her head, she mused to herself but loud enough that I heard, "My poor dear Mr. Chow. What'll I do?"

Then, turning toward me, she said, "You can use the phone in the kitchen."

"I'll use my cell phone. I have to go out to my truck since that's where the list of my clients' phone numbers is. I won't be long." *And it will give you time alone to consider the decision you must make.*

When I returned, I stopped at the drawer next to the sink to pull out a tea towel I'd noticed when I got the towel for the ice pack. It would make a sling for her arm.

I approached her with the cloth triangle and told her it would help stabilize her arm.

"Oh, no, you won't. My arm hurts too much to bend it and force it into a sling." Seeing that I was ready to protest and trying to appease me, she added, "It's okay. I'll be fine. I'll have my friend drive me."

"What's his number? I'll call."

"Never mind, Doctor! I'll take care of that in a few minutes."

Why is she so resistant? Guilt? Denial? What? I was frustrated. *No use arguing.* I learn slowly sometimes.

She shifted the ice pack from her shoulder down to her elbow. She seemed able to flex the fingers of her bitten hand.

I gave her a copy of the bill and handed her the pen and check-book she asked me to fetch off the kitchen counter. She had a difficult time holding the pen. She was left-handed. Bizarrely, a phrase I heard once popped into my head—"lefties are the only ones in their right minds"—but I wasn't sure about this case.

"It's okay. You can mail me a check later—when your arm is mended and you can write more easily."

Of course, she insisted on paying. "No, I'll just sit here. You go do *it* now." Yelling out to the patio, she cried, "Good-bye, Mr. Chow. I love you." She continued to struggle with the check. "Here you are," as she tore it out of the checkbook. "I want you to put Mr. Chow to sleep. I've decided," she said firmly. Pause. She winced. *Is her look from the emotional pain of losing her dog or from the physical pain of writing the check?*

"It's the wise choice," I assured her.

"Yes, I don't want any more bites." *Finally she used the word "bite!"* "Mr. Chow is just getting more and more vicious." Pause.

Thoughtful stare. "He really has been sweet." *Sweet? What sweet?* "He let me pet him." She paused again. "He let me pet him, but he wouldn't let me brush him much."

"I know you tried your best to care for him. Better take care of this now. So no one else gets hurt."

She agreed. "Don't let him wake up."

I glanced at the patio and heard the proverbial "sawing of logs" emanating from under the blanket.

"I'll be right back. Get what I need for the euthanasia. I'll need to know if you want a cremation and if you want his ashes returned."

"Will you take him? I want his ashes," she said quietly, staring off into space.

"Sure, I'll take him with me and see to the cremation." *She wants his ashes back! Well, I've canceled the rest of the appointments for today, so I might as well take him directly to the crematorium—once I take her for treatment at the ER and then drop her off back home.* I could be stubborn also. But I did realize my convictions might not be as strong as hers.

When I got back with my euthanasia kit, I had her sign the form giving consent to perform the task and have a private cremation.

I walked over to the snoring form under the blanket and shoved the head end with the toe of my shoe. No response. Walking back to get my bag, I asked her if she wanted to sit with him while I gave the injection. I was pretty sure he was still completely unconscious from the sedative. "I could help you to the chair on the patio." She declined. With an empty look on her face and her hand shaking, she signed the consent form.

I felt sad. For her.

I drew up more sedative into a syringe and approached Mr. Chow with caution and injected the dose into a muscle. A few minutes later I checked his level of sedation by poking his head once again with the toe of my shoe. No response. No snore. With my electric razor I shaved a hind leg to more easily see a vein. *Best inject into a vein in his rear—away from his head. You never know . . .*

After loading another syringe with the euthanasia solution (euphemistically called "pink juice" in the trade), I placed a tourniquet and then slid the needle into the large vein in his ankle area. Loosening the tourniquet, I pushed the plunger on the syringe. As is usual, because the solution is so thick, it took about half a minute to finish the injection. Breathing stopped within seconds. I took my stethoscope and listened for a heartbeat. None. He was gone.

I came inside and offered Ms. L. my sympathy. She thanked me again and insisted on giving me another check that included the additional services, which she laboriously wrote.

I still felt concerned, worried for her. *She needs the wounds dressed, X-rays, and antibiotics.* I wanted to scoop up her light frame and carry her to the truck to drive her to the hospital. But her protests were unquenchable as she adamantly turned down my offer. I extracted from her a promise that she would phone her friend for a ride. I handed her the phone and headed out back.

I lifted the now limp fifty-five pounds of Dog in the blanket to carry him to my truck. As I exited the side gate, she yelled out, "I love you. Mr. Chow, I love you."

I phoned that evening. I wanted to know how she was doing.

Still deflecting, she said, "Thank you so much for taking care of Mr. Chow for me. I really appreciate your caring."

"I wish I could have done more. What about you? What did the doctor say?"

I guess I should have anticipated her answer. "I'll go in the morning. I just want to take a hot shower. I took a pain pill I had from my last visit. I'll be all right."

"What? Oh, come on. I'll drive over and take you to Emergency right now. You need treatment, and . . ."

"And I'll be okay overnight. I'm stepping into the shower now. I want to finish and get into bed before the pill kicks in."

And what if it kicks in while you are still in the shower and you're woozy? You could slip and fall. I relayed my concerns to her, but it did as much good as a raincoat in the Sahara.

"Promise me you will call tomorrow and let me know how you are."

"Right after I get back from the doctor. I promise. I'll call for my ride first thing in the morning."

You haven't called yet?

"First thing in the morning. Good night. And thanks again for all your concern and help. I look forward to seeing you again when you bring my boy's ashes to me. Mr. Chow has been such a wonderful pet." Click.

The next two days were chock-full of appointments. During that time, I thought about how, when she went for treatment, the bite would need to be reported to public health and animal control authorities. I knew I could explain that it was a provoked bite, the need to euthanize right then and there, and that Mr. Chow did not have rabies.

The second night, while checking my voice mail, there was a message from Ms. L. "Hello, Doctor, I had X-rays. My shoulder bone is broken. Last night, I couldn't stand the pain any longer, so I took a taxi to the hospital. That was around midnight. At four in the morning, a nice nurse took me in for X-rays. They didn't do much, just gave me pills, put my arm in a sling, and told me to rest. Such an ordeal, but it'll heal. I'll be out of commission for a while.

Now don't you worry about me. Life is like that. Good-bye, and thank you again for helping my boy."

"Life is like that," she says. I could keep Mr. Chow from biting me and any more people but not from biting her. Then all I could think of was her saying, "He's never done that before."

6

Hey, You Forgot Something

Andrew and Savannah, two energetic Lhasa Apsos, yapped enthusiastically as I packed my bags of needles and vaccines—maybe glad to see me go after witnessing their feline roommates, Willie and Zoe, get poked and prodded. As I headed for the door, I was somewhat distracted as my mind was already on to the next house call.

As soon as I opened the front door and started to step out, both dogs glommed onto my pants, one on each leg, tugging with their teeth, their heads *Gr-r-r-r*ing from side to side.

I shook them loose, and Pat and I laughed at their shenanigans.

"Bye, Pat. See you next time." I waved, still chuckling.

"Keep well, Doc," she replied while closing the door as quickly as she could, holding the eager dogs back with her legs. It was autumn, and sycamore leaves were all over the yards in the neighborhood. The little rascals had been known to squeeze through any opening in the door to run off and play "jump and scatter the piles of raked leaves."

I drove to the end of the block and pulled over to the curb. I thought I would check my phone for voice messages before leaving for the next scheduled appointment. After all, I'd finished early with the cats. *Maybe I can squeeze in another appointment today.*

The voice mail chirped, "You have one new message." I checked. It was Pat calling to say the dogs were "fixed" at the front door.

I called her back. "Hi, Pat. What do you mean 'fixed'?"

"They haven't moved since you left. They're just staring at the front door, tails wagging, tilting their heads, listening. In total concentration, as if expecting something."

What?

She said, "Like expecting you back. I think you need to see them. You know they like you, and you only saw the cats. Maybe they just need some attention from you. You seemed a little distracted when you left."

Yeah, and tugging at my pant legs as if pulling me back should have gotten my attention.

On my previous visits, I had examined both dogs, regardless of which pet I was there to see. I always scratched them behind their ears and rubbed their bellies. But this day, I had rushed away in a determined efficiency mode.

When I arrived back and opened the door, I was immediately greeted with the usual enthusiasm. I bent down and patted the shaggy duo's wiggly bodies. They sniffed my hands all over, eagerly licking my fingers. They both hopped and twirled, barking and panting with tongues drooping out. I scratched behind their ears and rubbed their tummies as best I could considering how they kept sniffing my hands and dancing around.

Then it dawned on me. *Ah, I forgot.* I darted back to the car and pulled a bottle out of my bag. I slipped back inside the house to the chorus of barks.

As soon as I got the bottle out and shook it, they bounced up and down, mouths drooling in Pavlovian anticipation. I didn't give them their treat. I always hand them a chewable vitamin pill when I leave. But I didn't do it this time. I fed them the tasty tablets, and they immediately scampered off to the living room, jumped up on the couch, and began chewing their treats.

After I'd driven a half block away, I pulled over at the curb and called Pat on my cell. "How is your menagerie doing?"

"Willie and Zoe have gone into hiding, probably under the day-bed like they usually do. But, oh, the dogs. They are just as calm as could be. Right now, Andrew and Savannah are lying on the living room rug, contented from their chomping."

"Oh, good," I said. "Now there'll be peace in your household." *I won't forget their treats again!*

"Yes. And, you know, they even look like they have a grin on their faces."

7

The Maze

I stooped to pick up the *Sacramento Bee* newspaper on Mrs. Robin's porch. The porch light was on. As Mrs. Robin later told me in her best vocal rendition of Tom Bodett ending a Motel 6 commercial, "I always leave the welcoming light on."

As I rang the doorbell, remembrances of paper deliveries past paged through my mind. This house was on my route.

When the curtain of night would fall, early as it does in winter, I would deliver the *Bee* in the dark. I rode my bike through neighborhoods that even included the McClatchy city library, named after the publishing family that started the *Sacramento Bee*. At its peak, I delivered to 126 homes, my bicycle handlebars loaded with a canvas bag of papers. Since I lived in the middle of the neighborhood, I could deliver half of them, then return home and load up the rest.

There were two major newspapers back then in the 1950s. The *Union* was delivered to your doorstep before breakfast, so you could be up on the news before leaving for the day's activities. The *Bee* was delivered in the evening, for relaxing with the newspaper after work. I didn't like waking up early, so by default, I delivered the *Bee* after school.

It was fun, and I loved the challenge of flinging the rag from my bike as I rode by on the sidewalk, seeing how accurately I could plunk it onto the doormat without hitting the screen door. Or landing it in the bushes! One of my favorite customers would stand on the porch, and I would pitch the tightly folded paper to him. "Strike" he would call, waving his catch in the air as I rode by. It made my heart swell.

I was painfully shy as a kid. Not so now.

Despite my shyness, one of the highlights of my youthful job was to go door-to-door, collecting the monthly subscription fees. Back then, security was not the issue it is today, so some people openly left an envelope with cash in it on the doorstep or attached to their mailbox lid. Most of my customers answered the doorbell or my knock, and I would get to meet the people who lived behind the doors. Sometimes I got a glimpse into the interiors, which provided fodder for fantasies. Seeing the furnishings and surroundings, even in my youth, inspired imaginations of what their lives were like and what mysterious motives fueled them. The neighborhood was all middle class, but the people, in similar-appearing houses, were different, each unique and with a story of their own. That fascinated me then, as it does now. Most of my customers were very kind to this shy kid.

There is only one major newspaper now in Sacramento, the *Bee*, which switched to morning deliveries. Thankfully for my slow-to-wake-up body, I no longer work for them.

Serving that same neighborhood later, providing professional services to many of the same houses, brought on feelings of nostalgia and belonging. Perhaps it was the subconscious choice of returning to a home, a "hood" I felt comfortable with.

After Mrs. Robin and I exchanged greetings, I handed her the newspaper. She was short and thin, in her seventies, and wore a red-and-white checkered dress that reminded me of a picnic tablecloth. With a quick but choppy stride, she led me into the front room.

I told her of all the papers I had delivered to this house. Then I spotted them—neat rows in her "living room area." Piles and piles of newspapers stacked two to four feet high and in such a way that it made aisles, somewhat like the stacks in libraries. I shared my wonder of how many of the papers were delivered by me. But she assured me none in her stacks went through my hands, since she purchased the house a few years after I'd left and moved away to college.

She said her stacks provided all the knowledge and history anyone would have to know. She remembered articles from years ago. "Now I have something about that. Let's see, where is it?" She would rummage through a stack in the middle of one of the aisles and come up with an issue and rumple a few pages, opening the paper to the article she had in mind. This brought to my mind the house I grew up in, where our living room floor was littered with newspapers and magazines discarded by my prodigious reader (but underwhelming housekeeper) of a mom.

I saw the mounds of papers and magazines as a metaphor for Mrs. Robin's mind, as if all her memories were somehow there, stacked in neat, not so little piles, just waiting for a connection to be made.

Her tall, not so thin daughter walked into the room and introduced herself as Sylvia. She was dressed in a navy blue trouser suit, with a loose-fitting blouse that didn't quite camouflage her midriff fluff. After her mother left to search out Blackie, one of the feline patients I'd come to see, I talked in hushed tones about the stacks of newspapers. Sylvia informed me, "I know. I can't convince her otherwise. It seems a little touched, but she has her reasons."

"What might those reasons be?" Thoughts scrolled through my mind. *The cats are free—living among the newspaper maze.* I also thought of how cats could shred the papers for play or for litter material and thus soil their own living quarters. And I was thinking that, if any of her seven female cats were pregnant, they could shred the papers for nesting material in which to "queen" (have a litter of kittens). The thought crossed my mind that "litter" has more than one meaning in reference to cats—litters they give birth to and the litter in boxes they eliminate in. What an irony!

Sylvia continued, "At first, Mom kept the papers so she could look up articles later, when something came up. But her memory is not so good now. She used to have them stacked by date, but she no longer bothers with that. It's kind of her way of remembering things. It's as if she has it in a stack somewhere, it is still there."

"You mean the papers are her encyclopedia? Her library of events?"

"Kind of. Actually, it is more like a symbol of her memory. You know what I mean?"

"Yes, I think so," I said, as her mother walked out from the back bedroom and approached us.

"Blackie somehow got into my bedroom, under my bed. I tried to get her out, but I haven't been able to."

"Got a broom?" I said. "I can use that to get her out."

Cocking a suspicious eye, she said, "You won't hit her with it, will you?"

I laughed. "Not this time," I said with a wink. "Lots of my skittish patients have been under the bed or scurry away and hide there when I arrive at the house. I'll just get on one side and push the broom under the bed and slide it toward your kitty. My feline patients usually take flight and move to the opposite edge of the bed. That's where you'll be. When she comes your way, reach under, get hold of her, and pull her out. Or she may just scamper right up to your arms. Usually, just seeing the broom will excite a cat enough to move away from it and go to your side of the bed. But sometimes I have to nudge her with the broom and push her over to your side."

She fetched the broom and handed it to me. I beckoned Sylvia to come along. "We might need two of you to catch Blackie."

Mrs. Robin shook her head. "No, she won't come to my daughter, just me." So, the two of us, Mrs. Robin and I, marched to the bedroom.

Closing the door behind me, I said, "We don't want any of your other cats getting in here and sharing under-the-mattress space, nor do we want Blackie to escape."

I went around to the opposite side of the bed from the door and looked under. No Blackie that I could see. "Get ready," I told her. *It's dark under there; maybe I just can't see him. He is black after all.*

I swept the broom back and forth under the bed. But no cat came bounding out.

"Let's look in the closet. Sometimes they hide there. Sneaky little devils."

"Oh, that's not likely. I have too many piles of boxes and shoes in my closet. It's jammed full."

"Mrs. Robin, you'd be surprised where they can go. They can hide in the most unlikely places, I assure you. One day, I found one cat in a dryer and another cat under a washing machine, both at the same house! They are very adept at the hide-and-seek game." I added with a smile, "Being an appliance mover is one of the qualifications for being a house-call veterinarian who treats cats and other slithery creatures."

She raised her eyebrows and shook her head. We opened the door. Sure enough, there was a jungle jumble of items on the closet floor.

I started sorting through it all, parting hanging clothes as I did so. There were clothes that had fallen off their hangers, stacks of shoes, cardboard boxes of "keepsakes," more boxes of photographs and empty picture frames. Oh, and did I mention piles of shoes (to rival Imelda Marcos)?

Musky. A spilled perfume bottle lay on its side, its neck sticking out from underneath a shoe box. As I picked up the smelly box, out sprang a black cat. It scurried first to the door to get out. No luck there. It quickly turned and scuttled behind a TV cabinet in the corner of the room.

"It looks like we found him," I said excitedly.

She shook her head and peeked behind the cabinet, frowning. "How did you get in there, Spot? No, Doctor, that's not Blackie. Blackie doesn't have a white spot on her nose."

Retrieving the broom and leaning it against the cabinet, I laughed. "Well, at least we know where to find Spot when we get to vaccinating. Let's just leave her and the broom here. Now, where can Blackie be?"

I looked at the closet shelf.

"That's too high for a cat," Mrs. Robin said, just as I reached up to feel around there. Suddenly, a cat leaped down. Mrs. Robin's mouth gaped in complete surprise.

"It is amazing where they can get to. I had a closet-shelf cat once, too," I told her. "Rusty was extraordinarily shy of people. I got him from the Happy Tails cat rescue group. They have a no-kill policy, and so many cats needing a home. No one else would take Rusty because he wouldn't come up to you. But I'm partial to orange cats and understand shyness, so I took him in.

"The bottom shelf was about six feet off the floor, the next shelf about a foot above that. He would hide out all day on the top shelf of my closet. Then, at night, after I'd gone to bed, he would jump down and head for food in the kitchen and the litter box in the master bathroom. Then he would wander around the house meowing at the top of his lungs, not at all shy of being the 'town crier.' My other two cats seemed to be okay with it.

"But, as much as I liked Rusty getting down for a stroll, I had to close the bedroom door to muffle the noise so I could get some sleep.

"None of my clothes had ever appeared shredded from a cat clawing its way up. How Rusty got up to the shelves was a mystery to me until one night when I got out of bed to go to the bathroom. He was coming out of the bathroom, having just gone potty where I leave the litter box. I guess I startled him when I jumped out of bed with some urgency and stumbled toward him in my sleepy fog. He bounded across the room and leaped up the wall in the closet, scratching all the way up to the second shelf. There was a cross board on the side wall of the closet at about five feet high, which Rusty had no trouble at all bounding to in his first leap. I had screwed the board to the wall, intending to put a nail in it to hang up my robe. I never got to the nailing. But the next morning, I got to examining the wall. It was then I saw there were scratch marks on the cross board and on the edge of the first shelf where it abutted the wall. Mystery solved!

"Now let's solve the mystery of Blackie's hideout."

Mrs. Robin and I looked under the dresser, behind the dresser, under the TV stand, and behind it. Both sheltered hiding cats, Rufus, the dresser cat, and Spot—but no Blackie.

Then I spied a piece of cloth hanging down from the box spring on the door side of the bed. Yep, a tear. *Could she have gotten in there?* I got out a penlight and peeked under the bed. There was a swelling in the underside of the box spring's slipcover. *Could be.* The lump was too far to reach, so I took the broom and poked with the handle.

"Meow!" The lump moved.

"Ha, we've got her. Now, how to get her out?"

Good question. I asked Sylvia to come and lend a hand. "We'll stand the bed on its side, try to isolate her, or scare her to the tear in the slipcover." The three of us lifted the bed up to rest on its side, the cat meowing and moving among the spring coils. We had to lengthen the tear, but we eventually got Blackie out. We left the bed standing on edge. Mrs. Robin said she would repair the rip later.

The cats got examined, all fourteen of them (including the litter of five we found nestled in a cave scratched out in one of the arms of her newspaper maze). Those old enough received vaccinations. Mrs. Robin didn't know who the mother of the kittens was since the find was a surprise to her.

"I guess at least one of your males didn't get neutered." I told her of the health and practical reasons to get all of her cats "fixed." Her method of birth control was relying on fixing only the "men" (as she called them).

During the exams, I found that Rufus was still intact. The utility room was well lit, so I took care of that guy's surgery right then on the enamel top of the washing machine. I had the time since Mrs. Robin was my only scheduled house call for the day, and the anesthetic was short-acting. I didn't need the ultra-sterile environment of a hospital as there is no deep invasion of tissue with a feline castration. I made arrangements to spay her potential mommas the following week at a hospital at which I had surgery privileges.

Because of unsanitary conditions, such as the defecation on newspaper litter torn out of the maze, territorial marking of some corners of the piles by Rufus, and blood and uterine discharges on the "nest" in the one of the aisles, I tried to convince her to find other homes for some of her cats and to clean up the newspaper corridors and the floors. I knew the city was considering an ordinance to severely limit the number of pets that could be kept at home, and I didn't want that to become an issue for this lady who clearly loved and wanted the best for her cats.

I continued to see her brood for annual exams and booster shots for a few years. She cleaned things up and located homes for several of her cats. She found a way to fit a door and barricade in the hallway so that the cats were limited to the back half of the house. "I even found new places where the kitties go into hiding," she revealed.

She did reduce the area covered by the aisles of papers, saying she "rescued all the unsoiled newspapers." There were not so many aisles, but the aisles were stacked higher—high enough that the new memory lane would still be a maze to her grandchildren. Her filing system was intact. Now if only she could remember in which new stack the record she was looking for could be found.

Driving by her house on an early evening in late autumn, I saw a bunch of folded newspapers scattered about the front porch. Leaves from her sycamore tree covered the lawn. I stopped and got out of the car. The porch light was off. I pushed the papers aside with my foot, picking up the freshest looking one with the idea of handing it to Mrs. Robin when she came to the door. I rang the bell. I waited and rang again. No answer.

Looking around, I saw a man next door, raking leaves in his driveway. I approached, introduced myself, and asked about his neighbor lady. He told me her daughter came and got her. She moved a few weeks ago. He said her daughter told him that her mother was sick with dementia. "Her memory was failing."

8

A Dusting Off

"Curiosity killed the cat, but satisfaction brought it back" is one of my favorite expressions. It had to be the definition of my very first house call.

I was a brand-spanking-new doctor of veterinary medicine, having graduated in May 1966 from the University of California at Davis. I thought I knew everything.

The George W. Hooper Foundation for Medical Research hired me to be their vet on a research project dealing with wild animals and tropical diseases in the jungles of Malaysia. But before I could go, I needed training in handling viruses in the laboratory. They arranged for me to be tutored on Floor 15, the high-security bio lab of the research wing of the University of California Medical School, San Francisco campus.

My wife Anne, step-daughter, three-month old son, and I moved in with my aunt at her house on the Great Highway at Ocean Beach, San Francisco. I commuted to work by bus.

A laboratory assistant that I worked with, Doug, said his cat was acting strange. He asked if I would take a look at him. The signs—frequent squats over the litter box with little to show for it—convinced me that the cat must have cystitis (urinary infection). So I borrowed a sterile glass syringe and needle from the laboratory, loaded it with a quarter milliliter of Pen-G, a long-acting penicillin, and walked with him to his apartment during our lunch break.

He and his wife lived in a one-bedroom flat in a renovated Victorian a few blocks from campus. Sherri had lunch waiting. "But first," I said, "let's take a look at your kitty."

Spider, a short-haired gray tabby, was a neutered male that was overweight, common in cats with urinary bladder issues. I introduced myself by petting and scratching him behind the ears. I had my secret weapon, a piece of ground-up catnip I surreptitiously rubbed on his lower lip to distract him somewhat from my exam. As Spider licked and pawed at his chin, I held him by the scruff of the neck with one hand and palpated his abdomen with the other. Empty bladder. Since the bladder of pets with cystitis is irritated and feels full to them, the patients urinate often, but only a small amount at a time. *At least the bladder is not blocked. Spider can pee.*

I asked to see the litter box. "I want to check if there is blood in the urine." Clumping litter was not common back then, so it was easy to see whether the wet granular litter was pink-tinged.

"The litter box is under the kitchen sink," Sherri informed me.

One of the double doors under the sink had been removed for Spider to access the litter box. I was curious as to what was behind the other door—trash bin, I supposed. I crouched down and opened the door. Empty.

Rather than doing the logical thing of pulling the litter box out from under the sink, I crawled under. *No obvious blood on wet portions of the litter.* Taking a look around while under there, I could see above my head a couple of small, hinged doors fastened together by a brass clasp. *Curious. What is that for? Where does it lead to?*

I reached up and turned the clasp. The doors immediately swung down, I closed my eyes. Something was falling on me, dumping a bunch of "stuff" onto my face, neck, arms, and shirt. "What the?!" I sputtered, trying to shake off what had coated me.

I slid out and stood up. Flour and orange peels dropped off of me. I looked like a flocked Christmas tree or a doughnut dusted with powdered sugar and orange sprinkles.

Doug and Sherri were laughing their heads off. I continued to shake and brush off the dusting of flour, while they continued to laugh.

"What happened? Where did this stuff come from?"

Putting his hand up to his mouth to stifle a laugh, Doug said it was some garbage they put down the chute on the sink. He pointed to a four- to six-inch diameter hole in the top of the counter beside the sink. He said they scraped their trimmings into it. When it was full, they would hold a kitchen garbage bag underneath and open the doors to empty it.

"Good Lord. I've never seen such a thing."

Doug agreed, "Neither had I, but this apartment has one." As he tried to muffle his "tee hee" he handed me a wet kitchen towel for me to clean myself.

"At least there wasn't any leftover lemon meringue pie filling to scoop into it last night!" said Sherri with a burst of chuckling as she proceeded to clean up the mess under the sink and on the floor.

I was embarrassed. "Well, I guess that will teach me to ask first." My curiosity had gotten the best of me. But there was satisfaction in learning something new about "appliances" in old apartments.

I gave Spider the shot. He recovered. I didn't. They burst out laughing every time I visited their apartment after that, especially when I walked past the sink.

9

Gunshots in the South

In the early 1990s, when I was taking as many house calls as I could to build my practice, I made visits to most of the Sacramento region, including the south. My definition of South Sacramento was anything below the border of Broadway, an expansive boulevard of a street bisecting the city.

Now, that is an admittedly broad definition. Some of the neighborhoods were and still are defined by high population density, low income, and high crime. Other neighborhoods in that geographic description were and still are characterized by islands of nice pricey homes and quiet streets. I served both.

Gunshots were heard most nights in certain areas of South Sacramento. A high school classmate of mine, with whom I was still in contact and who lived down there, told me she and her husband had double locks on their doors. They said, "Gunshots at night are the rule," not the exception. They witnessed drug deals going down in broad daylight on their street corner. Newspaper headlines of gang shootings, home invasions, and robberies were common.

Pets, too, lived and were loved there.

There were clients in the South, such as Mr. and Mrs. Chandra, who fit the typical client profile of busy professionals with more than one pet. But little did I know how atypical the house call would end up being on this day.

Mr. and Mrs. Chandra, both schoolteachers, lived in an upscale house on the outskirts of the South Land Park area. Their home was close to Florin Road and in gang territory. It was the end of a lovely spring day at twilight, the time of no shadows. As I carried my satchel from my car to the front porch, I noticed three young men sitting side by side on a short retainer wall next to the steps. They eyed me up and down, noticing my medical bag and my doctor's smock. The fellow closest to me was whittling some object with his switchblade knife that he closed and flicked open as I passed by. He wore a cut-off T-shirt and long black jeans. The other two men sported heavy gold necklaces and wore nondescript short-sleeved shirts and khaki pants that reached to their mid-calf area. All three had slick black hair. The third guy was wearing a hairnet.

I was there on a routine visit to see the Chandras' two dogs.

Spot was a neutered male black border collie with a white chest and notable for a single oval white spot in the exact middle of the outside portion of each of his black ears. He was *her* dog, I was informed on my first visit a few years previous to this one.

Spot greeted me with his usual sharp bark. Border collies are a favorite working dog for sheep herders. As is true of his breed, he was high-energy and super alert. It did not escape Spot's notice when I took out my bottle of vitamin treats and laid it next to the vaccine vials I placed on the dining room table. He crouched all the way onto the floor next to the table looking attentively at the bottle as if it were a member of a sheep flock. I completed the exam kneeling on the floor. Spot didn't move an inch, his nose in the air pointing at the tabletop. I handed him a chewable vitamin tablet afterward. He swallowed it, hardly chewing or moving from his space. He wanted another. I relented. I called myself *Softy* (I love attentive dogs).

Spot's housemate, Penny, observed at a distance. She was a spayed purebred basenji hound—no spots, just a short, light brown haircoat with a collar of white fur, upcurled tail, and erect ears. She acted typical of dogs of that breed that I have had as patients—aloof, a curious but suspicious look in her eyes, as if I might not be worthy of her trust. She was barkless, a characteristic of the breed, but nevertheless tried to stand me off in her squeaky, raspy way. She would attempt to get away when I approached with the needle and syringe loaded with vaccine. As was the case on previous visits, Mrs. Chandra held Penny for me while Mr. Chandra stood in a relaxed casual stance nearby puffing on a burled briar pipe with a studious look on his face as he peered over his wire-rimmed eyeglasses giving detailed advice to his wife on how to restrain *his* dog.

Mrs. Chandra nodded in a *Yes, dear* manner and proceeded to hold *his* Penny in her own efficient way. Penny was no less fond of the tablet treat than was Spot, but she would have no part of my handing it to her. I had to place it on the throw rug and back away before she would hop in her characteristic way over and gently nibble at the treat before glomming on to it and wolfing it down.

The three of us chatted a few pleasantries. They were avid bird-watchers and excitedly told me about seeing a flock of phainopeplas settle momentarily in a pepper tree in their backyard that morning. They explained to me that they are the size and shape of cardinals or mockingbirds, and have a crest like cardinals. Their plumage was black or charcoal-colored. What made it so exciting for the Chandras was that this was the first time they had seen the species in the eighteen years they had lived in that house. Another checkmark in their bird book. They opened the book and proudly showed it to me. I looked over the long list of checkmarks. I admired their diligence and attention to detail and told them so. They were pleased and nodded to each other.

Before I left, I asked about the men lingering outside. "I haven't seen them before when I've come here."

Mr. Chandra replied, "I think those *cholos* are gang members. They loiter here every once in a while. We haven't had any trouble with them, but they make us nervous." Then, with what I swear was a worried look on his face, he added, "Just don't linger when you leave."

Now I too was nervous, and my hands began to feel clammy from sweat. Aware of seconds as if they were hours, I hurried down the eternity of the five porch steps to my car and quickly opened the trunk. I was lifting my bag into the trunk when the three men stood up and approached. The man with the knife rubbed it back and forth a couple of times on his jeans. He grinned and called out, "Hey, man, got a light?" He pulled a pack of cigarettes out of his back pocket.

It takes three of them to ask for a light? "Uh, sorry, no." I tossed my bag into the trunk.

The men kept sauntering toward me. I was sure they were up to no good. I could hesitate no longer.

Leaving no doubt about my motions, I swung my right arm in a wide theatrical arc around to my back and thrust my hand under my smock and stuck my fingers under my belt behind me. At the same time, I raised my left hand up and forward displaying my fingers in a halt signal. I said in a loud voice with as much low-register testosterone as I could muster, "Give me five!"

They stopped dead in their tracks. The lead guy put up a hand saying, "Okay, man. It's cool. Take it easy." Or something to that effect. He hesitated a moment and eyed me suspiciously before muttering a profanity in a low voice and backing away, still facing me. His followers slowly turned to walk the other way, their hands in front of them out of my sight. The knife-wielding man turned and followed.

I was shaking, wondering if one of them had a gun under his shirt and would pull it on me. Homicides were common in the area of South Sacramento over far lesser things than what drugs or cash I might have in my trunk. Fortunately, they settled back down on the concrete stoop they came from and watched. I felt like their eyes were throwing darts at me. I closed the trunk, hurried into the driver's seat, quickly locked the doors, and sped away.

Whew. Damn, that was scary. But it worked!

I had taken a concealed weapons course the previous year. I was not carrying my nine-millimeter Ruger pistol that day. Thank goodness I remembered the lesson and that the hoods knew what I was talking about and didn't doubt that I had a gun concealed under my smock. The instructor said that anyone who had done time in prison or hung out with people who had run-ins with the law would understand that "Give me five" means "Stand off and don't come any closer than five feet, or I will shoot you."

That was the last call of the day. I was done for anyway, still shaken, perspiring, and feeling the fear of *What if they didn't know what I meant or didn't believe I had a weapon?*

On the way home, I dropped in on a *Cheers*-like bar in my neighborhood. It was busy and noisy. *Good. I need to be in a crowd of "normal" people.* Happy laughter and reassuring jukebox music filled the air. I sat down on an empty bar stool, my shoulders sagging in relief. Waving to Miguel, the bartender, I shouted, "Vodka tonic. Double," and added, clearly, for good measure, *"por favor."*

In my view, the ails of the poor areas of cities are socioeconomic, with self-perpetuating cultural indulgences. It is not race nor ethnicity nor religion itself that lead to poverty. The behavioral norms established over time become ingrained in neighborhoods and lead to decay. Stereotypical behavior is often expected from those outside of that culture and often demanded by those trapped within.

"You're in a high-crime area, so you could be a criminal" can be the thought, even subconsciously. I was overtly guilty of that profiling when the three men approached me, asking for a light. It turned out that my assumption was likely right. But, they could actually have been honestly asking for a light, or maybe they were just curious about who I was and what I was doing in the area. I didn't give them the benefit of the doubt. It's always a touchy thing.

I had controlled substances in the cooler in the trunk of my car, drugs that had recreational street value far beyond their whole-sale cost to me. Veterinarians often use ketamine to induce rapid short-acting anesthesia. I had used it as an injectable cocktail mixed with other substances for heavy sedation, for example, for the quick surgery of a cat castration or a skin biopsy in cases where a patient was too squirmy and I couldn't hold the pet still enough for a local anesthetic to work. I no longer carry ketamine on house calls as there are now good alternative drugs that work as well for sedation and pain control.

I had a client, "L," offer to pay me handsomely for a vial of it. "Special K," "Super Acid," and "Cat Valium" are some of the terms used for it. The drug can distort vision and sound and give a feeling of detachment. L told me he snorted it occasionally at parties. He loved the feeling of being "out of body." He had the sensation of a Michael Jackson moonwalk six feet above the floor. Some of his friends felt the rush of a near-death experience. It has even been used as a date rape drug. Of course, I did not sell the drug to L. In fact, I "fired" him as a client. Thankfully, his cat appeared to be well treated and in good health.

Bolstered by the previous successful escape, I had another occasion to use the "five" technique.

It was a long day of short daylight in late November. Not yet wintery cold. A dreary moisture-laden overcast evening weighed oppressively on the leaden sky. I left home for my first house call in darkness and, after an unusually large number of appointments, was returning home in darkness, around 11:30 p.m. Low barometric pressure affects me, so I was feeling down with a mood that wasn't any brighter than the sky of the day. And I was hangdog tired.

I parked in the unit space assigned to my condo in the South Natomas area. The thought of a cozy bed awaiting me stirred my inertia. *Okay, get moving. The sooner you get going, the sooner you can drop your weary bones into dreamland and start sawin' logs.* I opened the car door, dropped my feet down to blacktop, stretched my arms in a waving movement, and shook my body head to toe to get circulation going. I trudged around to the back, opened the trunk, and removed my medical bag and cooler containing my pharmacy.

A huge man with broad shoulders, bulging muscles, and weighing I guessed over 220 pounds and standing about five-nine approached. I wore a light jacket; he didn't seem to mind the chill in his tank top, sporting mountainous biceps and pecs. His cutoff jeans showcased tree-trunk thighs. He was born pumping iron.

"How y'all doin', man?" Not really interested in my response, he continued, "Mah wife is havin' contractions. I gotta git her t' delivery room. Mah car won't start 'cause I got no gas." He paused, inhaling the cool air expanding his barrel chest. "Kin ya lend me ten? Jis fer gas, so I kin git help fer my poor woman 'n our baby."

There were so many panhandlers in the area. I'd seen him with his wife on the street not too long ago, and she didn't look pregnant. I was bushed. "Sorry. I just want to get up to bed."

His smile faded. He flexed his biceps. "I can crush a man's skull with these arms," flexing and mimicking squeezing a head like a watermelon between his barrel chest and his muscular arms. I could visualize it bursting its red pulp all over as it split apart in his vise-like motion. "Look, man, I don't want to hurt you. Give me ten. That's all I ask."

No way! My low-pressure feeling had me in a no-nonsense mood. Rising to the occasion, I stepped back, glowered at him, reached a hand under my smock behind my back and said, "And all *I* ask, man, is for you to Give Me Five!"

He laughed and said, "What the F you talkin 'bout? Yer nuts.' N I could crush those too." He stepped toward me, menacingly flexing ballooning biceps again. Right then, a car drove in the gate and headed toward my parking area. I crab-crawled toward the car. "Let's see if *he* has cash for you. I don't." (*Lie. Too much cash on me.*) I waved the car to stop and hand gestured that I'm okay and for him to roll down his window. At the same time, I called to him, "Witness," loud enough for both the driver and muscleman to hear.

Big biceps brute turned and ran off. *Whew!* The driver didn't roll down his window. He drove on past as if I wasn't there (maybe thinking *I* was a panhandler or a drunk). Anyway, as far as I was concerned, the driver rescued me from that clear and present danger.

Since the big guy lived somewhere in the neighborhood, the worrisome thought crossed my mind that I might encounter him again on the street.

As it turned out, I did see him again a few weeks later. He was walking in my direction on the same side of the street. I made sure I did not make eye contact with him. He walked right past, paying no attention to me. *Whew*, again.

I learned a good lesson from it. Just because someone looks like a thug and acts like a thug, doesn't mean they know a darn thing about the Give-Me-Five rule.

That wasn't the last time I was confronted with the possibility of violence.

Mr. Benjamin Miller was quite successful in the business of renting out storage units. He lived in a modest house in a small island of pricey homes that was surrounded by a sea of neighborhoods infested with the sharks of poverty. He greeted me at the front door and led me into his living room. I looked around. The furniture was comfortable, like the overstuffed leather couches seated in an L-shaped conversation arrangement. Though the room was not large, it was stylishly decorated. There were soft pastel rectangular carpets over dark hardwood floors. Carved wood sculptures, apparently obtained from travels abroad, perched on side tables and the long wooden chest under the front window. Hand-woven wall hangings were as common as paintings. Cozy and warm.

Miller had me drop by his house to interview me. "To see if I was the man for the job." Following his rather assertive and bossy manner of questioning me about my qualifications and how I would perform the procedure he had in mind, he informed me that I was "hired." I subsequently found out that I was recommended to him by one of my regular clients. The client told me he would have hired me simply based on her recommendation but was used to being a boss and acted a lot like he hosted the reality TV show *The Apprentice*.

Miller told me he wanted his dear midsized schnauzer, Sarah, put to sleep. She was old, not eating, and moved from place to place with stiff legs, stumbling, and sometimes falling over. Occasionally and more frequently, she would stand, stock-still, in one spot, staring into space—a sure sign of dementia. He informed me that I needed to be respectful of the ceremony that would take place during the preparation and injection of euthanasia and that I should leave immediately afterward. There was to be an afterlife ceremony. He and his friends would take care of Sarah's "remaining flesh" (as he put it).

The day arrived that I was to perform the task assigned to me by Miller. I pulled up to a street lined with parked cars. A space was left for me at the head of the driveway. It was a warm, late spring day, and the French doors at the side entrance to his house were wide open. I entered that way and almost had to shove myself through the crowd that had gathered for the ceremony. "Excuse me. Excuse me," I had to say several times to get to the couch where Sarah was lying.

There must have been twenty or more people squeezed into the relatively small living room. They stood in a semicircle, two to three deep, around the couch. There were lit candles in glass holders on furniture and windowsills all around the room. Some being held by women, none by men.

Sarah was lying on her right side at the corner of the couch with her eyes closed and her nose pointing toward the edge. Her coat was dull gray, no longer a schnauzer silver. Mr. Miller was crouched on the floor beside her. He wore a skullcap, a white long-sleeved button-down-collar shirt with a black bow tie, and a pair of black slacks. His shoes, I noticed, by contrast, were a scuffed brown that matched the color of his cap. (*Purposeful?* He had seemed like such a detailed and fastidious person during my interview.)

Without rising, he greeted, "Dr. MacVean, so glad you are on time. Just in time. What I need you to do is kneel down beside me, do the good death as quickly as you can, and then leave." He had paid in advance by mail a week before the appointment. "My friends and I will conclude a brief ceremony before you give the injection." He did not smile nor look sad. He was not unfriendly, just intent on carrying out his plan.

"Okay, I'd like to access the brachial vein in her right leg."

"No, I don't want to turn her over. Use the left leg."

I understood how he didn't want to disturb Sarah by moving her. At the same time, I was thinking that the angle of needle insertion would not be as easy the way Sarah was laying.

I wanted to pet her and say hello and something like "such a pretty girl." But it was clear from Miller's expression and from the immediate beginning of the ceremony that there was no time for interaction. *Just get on with it.*

The circle of people closed tighter. A man, dressed casually but with a beaded scarf around his neck and a skullcap on his head, inched forward holding a small book (Torah? I wondered). He began to chant a short prayer.

As I opened my bag to take out the bottle of euthanasia solution, needle, and syringe, I looked around at the crowd: white, black, Hispanic, Asian, a few of each, a real salad bowl of culture. Most were dressed casually, only a couple of men in sport coats. Many of the men wore short-sleeved shirts and jeans, some with cutoffs.

The women were more noticeable in their dress. Some women wore sexy slim dresses with low-cut necklines. A couple of women wore loose-fitting dresses of thin textiles that draped loosely over their bodies. The jagged hems reminded me of pictures I'd seen of the habit of a witch's coven. They swayed back and forth.

Miller leaned over Sarah, mumbling something to her that sounded like Hebrew (not that I knew for sure what Hebrew sounded like). The crowd started to chant in a way that lent a mystical, even occult, quality to the ritual. I figured it was possibly a cobbled-together Kabalistic ceremony or some syncretic adaptation.

As I was drawing the solution into the syringe, someone knocked into my back and caused me to lose my balance and fall forward toward the couch. Instinctively, I pushed back. As I turned around I was faced with an angry young man who was drawing a deadly looking switchblade knife.

He yelled as he flicked the steel open and sharply waved it at me, "Don't touch me, man. Nobody touches me." His nostrils flared. Stunned silence sliced the room.

Geez. What the . . . ? His actions were so out of proportion.

Quickly, and decisively, Miller jumped up and yelled at the man. "Whoa, stop it. You crazy? He did nothing. Cool down. Back off." He then brushed the back of his hand across the man's chest in a friendly manner.

I fired off, "Listen. I need room. I can't have someone pushing me while I'm carrying a needle. I need to kneel down and give an injection. I need room to do this. Otherwise, I stop right now." I was assertive, but my hand was starting to shake. I began to perspire. It was not a hot day, but it suddenly was a sizzling room. I wondered why the guy was so touchy about my pushing since he was already crowded by others in the tight circle.

To me, Miller assured, "It's okay. No one means any harm. Please proceed. We can finish the ceremony after you leave. Please." Then to everyone else, especially the knife-wielder, "Now everybody just settle down. Give Doc some room. Remember, this is for Sarah."

A breathy sigh of relief seemed to fall from the crowd.

Miller knelt back down to Sarah, stroked her head, and nodded to me to go ahead. I took a deep breath, got down beside Sarah, and applied the tourniquet. When I removed the cap of the hypodermic needle and bent over to insert the point into the vein, it seemed like the circle backed away a little.

After the injection was over and I'd given my condolences to Mr. Miller, I picked up my bag and turned to the circle. "And my sympathy to all of you here to share in Sarah's passing." A faint smile appeared on several faces, and the circle widened and opened up an aisle for me out to the doorway.

As I walked past the crowd, the knife man patted my back. "I'm sorry," he said. Others voiced, "Thank you." I heard one lady whisper, "Namaste."

I could hear more chanting and low singing as I entered my car. No, not a typical house call at all. Again.

In the poor areas of Sacramento there are residents who don't have automobiles and would call me out for a vet visit. Although appearing poor, they seemed to have money to pay for the house call. In fact, they were often willing to give their last dollar for their precious pet.

Occasionally, I did get stiffed on my fee and my time. But only when their pet was a dog. It was never a cat. Admittedly, it's only a small sample upon which I base my conclusion that people who are going to take advantage will do so for a dog. Maybe, to them, a cat isn't worth the effort. I love cats, so it is sad that cats are undervalued.

Oak Park has very recently risen like the phoenix and is now an upcoming desirable place to live in Sacramento. In the decade after World War II ended, that area south of Broadway was a nice residential and light commercial place. Many times, we kids, my sis and I, would ride our bicycles from our home on 24th and W streets, cross Broadway, and enjoy hot summer days swimming in the Oak Park community pool. The houses were old, some were Victorian ladies. But over the following couple of decades, decay and the putrefaction of drugs and prostitution took its soul.

It was in a run-down, poor area in Oak Park that I met Brutus. He was a snarling, drooling, ready-to-rip-my-head-off, 140-pound Rottweiler. A tall, thin man wearing a tattered denim jacket and jeans met me at the door of his small, sagging shack. He was around forty years old with skin of obsidian that reflected his hard, dark nature and called himself "Smith." He claimed to be the dog's caretaker as he stepped out on the minute, concrete pad that pretended to be a porch and closed the door quickly behind him to keep the barking beast at bay.

He had a broad, cruel grin that showed a gap in dentures from a missing upper incisor tooth. One tooth next to the dark cave was a dentine stalactite with a shiny gold crown. I had quoted a price range over the phone when Smith called. He said he wanted the cheapest possible treatment. It was before Christmas. "I need a little left for gifts," he informed me.

He said Brutus had a festering "dawg" bite. My job would be to lance and flush the abscess and give an antibiotic shot. Of course, I had to muzzle him. I wasn't about to get close enough to place the muzzle over his lips that curled up into a snarl and displayed large sharp fangs as he faced me. My intent was to illustrate to Brutus's human companion how to apply the muzzle by using hand gestures and placing the large plastic cage-type muzzle over my face. I did that, including even encircling the straps around my head, under my ears, and fastening the buckle tightly behind my neck.

Laughing, he said, "Y'all look like they put ya in th' mask that was on th' crazy guy in that movie. Wha was . . . *Silence of the Lambs.*"

I had to laugh at that also. "Do you think you can get this on Brutus? It'll need to be very snug. Buckle it tight. And we'll need to keep him from pawing at it, trying to brush the muzzle off. We'll also need a leash to hold him in place." Looking at this skinny, actually frail-looking man I wondered if he could restrain Brutus enough. I had figurative fingers crossed in my mind.

The man said he would fetch his "woman," as he called her when he didn't call her "bitch." He opened the door a crack and yelled to somewhere inside the house. "Get your fat ass out here and help hold the rope, damn it." She was in her early twenties, had a pretty face, was short, a little plump but muscular. She wore a plain dress that hugged her figure. Her olive skin was smooth and shiny. *What is an attractive woman like her doing with a man like that?* She held out a good-sized rope. He grabbed the rope, smiled at me, took the muzzle out of my hand, and started to go inside to attend to Brutus.

"Hey, Smith, hold on. I have a collar and leash in my car. It'll be a lot easier than your rope. You can use that."

Looking at me like I must have a screw loose, he declared, "Ah never put a collar on m' dog before, n' I never will. Dogs are meant to guard, not be pussied around."

It was beginning to dawn on me that maybe it was a mistake to take this call. *You think?* There was clearly no training this crude guy. I just hoped he was savvy enough to get that muzzle taut.

Smith grabbed his woman by the arm and started to push her toward the door. "C'mon, bitch." She shrugged, pulled her arm loose, and stood there in silence. She shed his sarcastic mutterings like a chow dog shedding its undercoat in summer.

Finally, he opened the door for her, and they both went inside. The door slammed shut. I heard yelling and scuffling going on. But soon the door opened and out came Smith, his woman, and Brutus growling between them. The muzzle was on, and the rope was held firmly up close to the neck. I reached over and checked. The straps were buckled tight. *Whew, now what?*

"Okay, looks good. Let's go inside and get it done." I picked up my bag and started for the door.

"Where you goin'?"

"We'll go inside where it's warmer and get some hot water running and a towel to wash up . . ."

"Nope. Gotta do it outside while they's still light. And there ain't no hot water. F***ing P.G.&E. cut off th"lectricity."

Uh, oh! Shoot. It's cold out here. All right, Duncan, just get the job over with. I turned up the collar on my smock. To the woman, I asked what her name was. She said it was Beth. *Much better than his "B" word.* I then asked her, "Please, Beth, can you get a pan of water and a towel?"

With that, Beth ducked inside and fetched a pail with cold water and a washcloth. To my surprise, thin-man Smith was able to hold Brutus without the woman's strong hands.

"Okay. How will we keep him in place while I treat him?" I mumbled to myself as I looked around the yard. No lawn, just dirt. Actually mud from rain the night before. Not good sanitation. It wasn't ideal. *Ideal? What's ideal got to do with it?*

I spotted a chain-link fence with a gate on the side of the house. "Bring Brutus over here. We'll feed the rope through the fence and back through near his rear end, wrap the rope around his body and under his belly near his hind legs, and then thread it back through the fence. Beth, you get inside the gate and hold the loose end of the rope tight. Smith, you help hold his neck against the fence and keep his front legs from pawing at the muzzle. Okay?"

They were puzzled but complied. Fortunately, after he was trussed up, Brutus didn't struggle much at all.

"That's it. We can do this." I sloshed through the mud over to the "porch" to get a scalpel and blade, forceps, a syringe of antibiotic, an alcohol spray bottle, and gauze pads. I stuffed them in my pockets and carried the water pail and cloth back to the patient. There was a puncture wound on his upper thigh, but no pus oozed out when I squeezed it. The skin immediately next to the hole was bulging. I probed the hole with the alligator-like prongs of the forceps to see if there was an embedded foreign object. I wasn't at all sure it was a dog bite that caused the wound. *Bullet? A sharp piece of wood? Wrong time of year for a foxtail.* The probing came up empty.

After washing the bulging skin next to the hole and spraying with alcohol, I made a quick stab into the bulge. Out poured bloody pus. No anesthetic, since the quick entry of the sharp surgical blade wouldn't hurt any more than rapidly ripping a Band-Aid off. I pressed the area around the bulge until no more fluid ran out.

A forceps probe of that pocket of pus was negative also. I washed the area again and gave a long-acting antibiotic shot into the thigh muscle.

Patting Brutus on the rear, I announced, "Done. There it is. Good job holding."

They both smiled proudly. After unwinding the rope, they took Brutus to the door, stopping long enough to undo the muzzle and hand it to me. Smith patted his dog on the head and said, "Good boy. Good dog. You're my man." Brutus got one more growl in before he disappeared inside. Smith said he would get the "cash payment," as he put it.

I washed up and placed the dirty instruments in a plastic wrap. I carried the supplies and medical bag out to the car. I was thinking that he treated his dog better than he treated his woman.

After a few minutes, Smith came outside. He was smiling from ear to ear yet managing to hold a lit cigarette between his lips in the gap in his dentition. The tobacco tube bobbed up and down as he spoke. "Gotta hand it to ya. Thanks." Then he forked over a wad of bills.

While I was starting to count the cash, I asked, "How did it happen? Where's the other dog that bit him? I guess the attacker got away unharmed?" My suspicions of causation by something other than a tooth had been aroused. *Is there more to the story that he might be hiding?*

Smith took a drag on the cig and mumbled something about no other dog in his house. Then he said more loudly, "Gotta go. God bless." He turned to go back into the house.

By then I noticed he had given me only five ones, a five, and a tenner. I had quoted him $90, which was less than a normal fee since I tried to give the poor man a break. I shook my head in disbelief. "No, it's ninety."

"But all I gots is twenty dollahs."

"You think a doctor's time and treatment is worth only twenty bucks? What if your boss where you work gave you a mere dollar for every hour worked? What are you thinking?"

"Cash. All I got." He turned his pockets inside out. Empty.

He shrugged his shoulders and turned to go. With sarcasm I snarled back, "Well, now you'll have money for Christmas. Merry Christmas."

I battled the urge to grab him and give him more of my mind. I even imagined pushing him to the ground, getting a dental extractor out of my bag, and pulling his gold tooth as payment. Then I thought of the arrest for assault and battery that would follow. *Scratch that idea.* It was futile. What could I do? Take him to small claims court? That would be a waste of time and money.

I was disgruntled the rest of the day. The deliberate rip-off. He knew what he was doing and that he would get away with it.

Getting shorted of cash happened a couple of other times. Then there were the house calls where I arrived only to find no one home. No-shows and wasted time. In three other instances, the people inside their house refused to answer the door. *Then why did you call me in the first place?*

To make it clear, there were times even in more well-off areas of town that shorting occurred. Bounced checks were the most common in the more affluent areas. Some were intentional, and some were not. I learned, not as quickly as I should have, to recognize those situations and to charge a fee for checks returned because of "insufficient funds" (as the bank called it). It was never really about the money. For me, it was the insult and the wasted time. Truthfully though, after I got over my initial anger, I was able to rationalize that the time wasn't actually wasted. I did some good. A pet in need got treated.

These events occurred early in my house-call fee-for-service career. I tried to smile at my minor misfortunes and tell myself that they were simply business lessons learned. But I did make a decision regarding those lessons. Since I did not live in the South area, I decided to stop going down there. There were two other competent veterinarians who did house calls and who lived in or near the area. I admired their apparent ability to deal with those clients, perhaps better than I could. I referred most of the would-be clients in the South to those doctors.

There were occasions I forayed into South Sac to serve a loyal client and their beloved animal companions, but those visits became rare as time passed by.

No more visits to gunshot alley.

10

Houses on the River

There was this pug, Maggie, whose eye had popped out.

Her caretaker lived in a houseboat that was temporarily anchored at the shoreline, down from the embankment of Miller Park, on the Sacramento River, south of the main part of downtown. I parked up top, putting my business card on display in the window of my car, hoping that might keep me from receiving a ticket for not paying a "day-use" fee.

Mr. Sanders ("Please call me Tom") was a short, stocky man with a round face, salt-and-pepper beard, and a ruddy complexion. His hands were round like his face, his fingers short and fat but strong. It was tough to match his grip when we shook hands. His age was obscure to me. I couldn't discern if his rough, ruddy skin was born of the sun and wind or due to the passage of time.

Soon after the pleasantries of greeting and being invited to have a chair at a worn, wooden desk in a corner near a potbellied stove, I started to fill in details for my record. Maggie settled in next to my pants leg, wagging her little curled tail and licking my hand when I leaned over to pet her. She ignored her eye as if it was a most natural thing to have an eyeball leaning out of its socket.

"How old is Maggie?" He didn't know.

Ignoring the popped-out eye for now, I examined Maggie. She had a shallow groove on the outside edge of her lower canine teeth and matching grooves on the inside of her upper canines. Her jaws were in alignment (not always the case in short-nosed breeds such as the pug). This wearing of enamel from teeth rubbing against each other over time indicated she was at least seven years of age.

"Is she spayed?" He didn't know. I felt tight little bundles of tissue under the skin, scarring from sutures, and saw the white line of a former incision on Maggie's abdomen. The surgery was likely the sterilization of spaying.

While I finished conducting the physical exam, Tom told me about Maggie's jobs—being a good companion and chasing birds off his deck so he wouldn't have so many droppings to clean up. *A zealous guardian.*

Eschewing full anesthesia, I gave a sedative cocktail by injection in a back muscle (faster absorption into her bloodstream than by injection into the thigh).

Some breeds of dogs have naturally bulgy eyes, which are a result of shallow eye sockets. Pugs are one of them. The congenital protrusion can make these dogs predisposed to the eyeball popping out of the eye socket. The most common cause of this is trauma, but sometimes the cause is unknown.

Maggie's right eyeball was extruding out of the bony eye socket but was not dangling by a cord of muscle and optic nerve as sometimes occurs with severe trauma. There was no exterior bleeding, but there were a few tiny red plaques under the surface of the white part of the eyeball, suggesting rupture of some small veins due to pressure when the eye popped out or due to blunt trauma to the eye. There was no swelling in the eyelids or surrounding tissue, which might suggest bruising and edema from a blow to the head. Also there was no swelling of tissue that might suggest a tumor growing from behind the eye that could cause the eyeball to prolapse.

"Tom," I asked, "do you know of some injury to Maggie's head that might have happened?"

Tom had a sheepish look on his face when he answered. "Uh, well, uh, Maggie did fall overboard when I dropped a hanging flowerpot I was watering. It was when I fished her out of the drink that I noticed the eye wasn't right."

I didn't think hitting the water could do the damage, unless she landed headfirst on floating debris, such as a log or other floating detritus. "Was she underfoot? Could the pot have bounced off her head?"

"Uh, I guess so." He still had that look that might have belied guilt from carelessness of dropping the pot on Maggie's head. Anyway, that's how I interpreted it.

The condition was minor and, in my assessment, did not require surgery. Maggie was such a cooperative patient. She probably didn't even need the sedative, but my rationale was that it would calm her, and the drug did have some ameliorative effect on pain. Washing the eye with saline flushed the surface dirt and mucus off. I tugged on a sterile surgical glove. The next step was simply applying firm, steadily increasing pressure with my gloved hand as evenly as possible over the surface of the eyeball. Then, pop, it was back in place.

Tom couldn't look while I pushed the eye in. So he talked about the weather and the fact that there wasn't too much debris floating along the river. He commented that sometimes flotsam and broken trees that float downstream make navigating difficult for his houseboat. Tom said he didn't know when the last vaccination boosters were given. "But I think she did have her shots."

While I was washing my hands in the bowl he called his kitchen sink, I saw a piece of paper lying on a side table. The letterhead read, *Dr. Dean Mattleboard, N.D. (Naturopath).*

"I remember this guy," I said, pointing to the paper. He lived along Garden Highway in one of the houses built on stilts at the edge of the Sacramento River. The doctor wasn't at home when I made my house call there, but his wife was. She was strung out on drugs, I thought. She had that meth look—thin, skinny actually, with under-eye shadows and prominent cheek bones. Her lips curled in like those of people with no teeth or like she was sucking on a lemon. Her movements were jerky, and her speech choppy. She had a dog named "Maggie"—*the same one?*

I asked Tom about it. He answered, "Yes, Theresa was my daughter."

Was? "Oh, gosh, I'm really sorry. Forgive my intrusion." I felt bad also because I'd given out some doctor-client privileged information.

There were no tears in his eyes, but his lids sagged with sadness. "That's okay." Shaking his head, he continued, "She's disappeared. The next-door neighbor realized after a few days had passed how unusual it was that she had not seen either my daughter or son-in-law coming or going. Theresa was always on the go, so it was odd that her car in the driveway had not moved.

"The neighbor went over there and knocked on the door. She tried the knob, but it was locked. She was worried since she had heard a lot of banging and shouting a few nights before. The other two cars that were there that night—the doctor's SUV and someone else's red Corvette—were gone the next morning. The house became silent after that; nothing stirred. She told me her hair stood on end as she peered inside the vertical window beside the front door, so she followed her intuition and phoned the sheriff's office."

"It must have been hard for you once you heard the news."

He cleared his throat. "They found a trace of what was later determined to be Theresa's blood on a sheet on the bed in a small basement room." I had seen the room when I made my house call there. It was more like a closet, crowded, only a twin bed, small nightstand, and space heater. "Drug paraphernalia were on the table. Traces of methamphetamine were found."

Tom dabbed at the corners of his eyes with a handkerchief.

I felt uneasy asking for more details of the story that was clearly still heavy on his heart. I told him I thought I recognized having seen Maggie before because of the way her left ear sagged more than her right ear and had a large black spot that covered the top half of the ear.

Tom gazed out through the back door, maybe upon the river as if it were a memory flowing by. A horn honked up above, somewhere in the parking lot. He blinked and turned to look at me. He continued his story, while I wondered if that honk was notification from a parking attendant that I was ticketed. *Well, I can't go check now. Can't leave in the middle of his misery.* I felt bad that I'd turned my attention away from him to a stupid ol' ticket.

"A deputy rousted me from my bunk on a friend's barge that was anchored at Ridley. I was hungover, so I wasn't much help. They asked me a lot of questions about the comings and goings of Theresa and her husband and who their friends were. I couldn't tell them much. They were interested in the fact that I had witnessed shouting matches between the two of them and that I never saw him ever hit or push her. Quite the opposite, she would throw things at him and slam her fists into him. She would be quiet as a mouse and then suddenly flare up into a rage."

He walked over to his desk, opened a drawer, and pulled out a photo. He handed it to me. "This was taken after she graduated from UCLA." It was a beaming father and daughter, arms around each other.

"What a great photo. She looks so radiant. She's gorgeous." Thinking of him, I added, "And you're not so bad-looking yourself."

"Was. We both went downhill after that."

I tried to interrupt and negate that impression, but he went on. "No, she started losing her looks after marriage and wild parties. Her husband, the doctor, always looked the same—handsome, controlled, a persuasive talker. She just loved to have fun." He brushed a hand over his beard. "Until the fights started. The drugs, the lowlifes who were sometimes there at Theresa's invitation. I quit stopping at their dock. It wasn't good anymore."

A pause, another swipe of his beard. "She's never been found. Some witnesses have insisted they've seen her in run-down areas of San Francisco, Seattle, and Miami. I don't know what to believe. The cops have never been able to pin anything on the doctor or his girlfriend with the red Corvette, although they still remain 'persons of interest.'"

I felt bad. I put my hand on his shoulder. "How sad. I'm so sorry for all that." I couldn't think of anything else to say at that moment. I felt inadequate to the event. I squeezed my hand on his shoulder.

He shrugged, straightened up, and inhaled deeply. He shook his head. "That's life. Sometimes. No end." Taking another deep breath and stepping toward the kitchen sink, he asked, "Can I fix you a drink? I need one."

"Sure. A glass of water will do." I wanted a shot from the Maker's Mark bottle that was sitting on the counter in front of his hand, but I still had a couple of calls to make.

He got out two glasses. He filled one with the bourbon, neat. He handed the other glass to me and pointed to the cask of bottled water at the end of the counter. I filled my glass and took a long drink.

After downing a couple of sips from his glass, he said, "Let's get on with Maggie."

Oh, yeah, Maggie. I looked around and found her out on the bow, sitting on the deck licking up some leftovers from fish cleaning. I picked her up and carried her into the parlor. Her breath smelled fishy. I sat in a chair at the small desk up against a wall, holding Maggie in my lap, scratching behind her ears. She lay quietly on my lap like a pudgy rag doll. With her saggy forehead skin and droopy ears and wrinkled skin over her short nose, she looked sad. But her licking my hand and wagging her tail and snuggling

88

close up against my belly told me she forgave me for pushing on her eyeball.

Tom was rummaging through a cardboard box. He pulled out a folder and handed it to me. It was labeled MAGGIE. "This was given to me by my daughter the last time I saw her. She asked me to take Maggie while she 'got herself straight.' I don't know what else is in the box. It's too sad to go through it. I'm just storing it for Theresa."

Just storing it for her? Then he has hopes for her return! Hope, that captive that keeps you eternally on the lookout for something, if only out of the corner of your eye.

I opened the file and saw that it was Maggie's records, including a receipt from the last time I had visited to give her shots, three years ago. *Three years, not long. Maybe there is hope.*

"It looks like all the shots are overdue, but just. We'll catch her up right now, Tom, so don't worry." *Don't worry? Where did that come from?* I'm not sure what I was thinking, but I remember the thought vividly.

I lifted Maggie off my lap and gave her the vaccinations.

I also noticed on that receipt that I'd given Theresa's two cats vaccinations the same day. I asked about them. "What became of her cats, Sly and Kit?"

"She said they disappeared during one of the fights she and her husband had. The doctor hated the cats. He once told me he hated Maggie, too. He said Maggie was a walking 'allergy.' Theresa thought he was allergic to Maggie—but also to everything else, including herself and anything she had to say."

The air felt leaden again, so I started chatting. You know, light things. I asked if he lived permanently on the houseboat.

He said he did. Not in Rio Vista, where he picked up his mail, but at various places along the Sacramento River Delta. He laughed and said he was a "river rat." I knew what he meant since my sister often sailed her boat up and down the Delta. She told me stories of the partiers who developed camaraderie at floating bars and at docks and at anchor along the byways.

I asked him why he was anchored here on the river edge of Miller Park instead of at the marina along the embankment on the other side of the river. He said he didn't want to pay the overnight fee at the "swanky yacht club." He'd rather just anchor out by the park and, for a change of venue, cook a hot dog or steak up at a barbeque pit in the park. "It is pretty," he said.

Miller Park, an area I knew well. I used to ride my bicycle from my childhood home at 24th and W Streets to the levee of that milk-chocolate-colored river, right at the end of Broadway. In summer, I would fish from the shore—mostly catfish, striper, shad, and occasional black bass. Though I tried, I never did catch a salmon there when they were running. The bank where I stood was muddy and slippery, so I had to be careful when leaning over to bring in my catch. There was no rocky bank nor gentle slope nor nearby boat dock like there is now. Oh, those lazy vacation days of childhood summer.

The park is pretty, as Tom said, but not always quiet since it's popular for evening family gatherings. He said he sometimes joined the families, even feeling a part of some "familia." "And the park rangers don't bug me. They let me anchor overnight. I never overextend my stay." Then he added one of my favorite proverbs, "Guests, like fish, stink after three days."

We laughed. Whew, the leaden weight had melted.

I finished the vaccinations, and he asked if Maggie's eye would be okay now.

"Yep, should be fine. Just a freak accident. Don't need to suture it in place, unless it occurs repeatedly. Sometimes we have to remove the eye completely if it pops out too often or too far out or is damaged too much. But I don't think anything like that will be for Maggie. Also, in my experience, most dogs retain normal vision after such a minor prolapse."

Tom added, "Maggie's a tough dog."

"Well, now that Maggie is a shipboard dog, maybe you should call your dog Popeye." Then, singing, I added, "Popeye the sailor man. Toot. Toot."

Tom chuckled and protested, "But she's Maggie, not Max!"

"Okay, then how about Olive Oyl?"

People tell me things. Unbidden. Sometimes I'm just too nosy. Sometimes I listen too long. I left the house call late for my next appointment. After a few blocks, I slowed and pulled over to the curb. *They'll find her, I'm sure.* My heart twinged. I can't help it.

II
Bats, Rats, and Lizards, Oh My

"The best thing about animals is that they don't talk much."
—Thorton Wilder

"Eye of newt, and toe of frog,
Wool of bat, and tongue of dog,
Adder's fork, and blind-worm's sting,
Lizard's leg, and owlet's wing . . ."
—William Shakespeare, *Macbeth*

"Dogs look up to you, cats look down on you. Give me a pig! He looks you in the eye and treats you as an equal."
—Winston Churchill

11

Mr. Black

On the outside, the house was a bright and cheery buttercup yellow with white trim. The sidewalk up to the porch was swept clean. The white door was inviting, as were the colorful red geranium flower beds on both sides of the narrow porch. Off to the right, there was a window well. A hint of what was to come was the deep black of the basement windowpanes.

Satchel in hand, I rang the doorbell. A minute went by. No answer. I rang again. *Wait.* Then I heard a shuffling and a tapping coming from inside the wall to the right of the door. *Ah, someone is coming.*

A cough, a sliding latch, and the door swung inward, and light poured into the hall and splashed on lines of tropical colors on a rectangular throw rug. The man-boy standing before me was tall, maybe six-feet-something. He was thin, with sunken cheeks, and stood pencil straight, his torso enclosed in a black linen tunic. Black denim trousers ended in a cuff at the top of dulled black leather shoes.

His voice cracked, "Hello, Dr. MacVean?"

I wondered if he was as young as his voice, which suggested the hoarseness and cracking of a teenage boy. He appeared more like he was in his early twenties. I looked into his dark and deep eyes. His curly black hair looked dyed. The eyebrows certainly were.

"Hi, and you must be Leonard Black. Good to meet you," I replied, extending my hand.

He shook my hand. His skin felt thin, like tissue paper, but warm to the touch, belying the cold-white boniness of his fingers. In fact, all of his exposed skin was so pale, I imagined he hadn't seen the light of day for some time. "I'm very glad you could be here on such short notice. I didn't think anyone would come today. I did call another house-call doctor, but he didn't want to come."

Curious use of words, "didn't want to come."

He continued, "You answered my phone call so expeditiously. Thank you."

He doesn't talk like a teenager. "Expeditiously" indeed. Have to find out his story.

Last night, I had arrived home from a movie with a friend and decided to check my answering machine for messages before heading to bed. It was nearly midnight, and the blinking of the red light on the machine always nudged my curiosity. One never knows what will come in next. The variety of my practice keeps me intrigued and always wondering what patient problem and what people I will meet next. The light indicated a message, one, which came in at 11:10 p.m. "Please call. My . . . ," the voice choked up with a cough. He did manage to leave his telephone number and name. It sounded strange; it came in late. *Might be an emergency.* I called back, got his address, and arranged to meet him around 10:00 a.m. I was excited by the call and imagined it would be an interesting visit. I love challenges. My adrenaline jumped, and I barely slept.

But this guy, this Mr. Black, had my attention today.

"This is my mom and dad's house." *Ah, explains the colors of the house, so different from the appearance of Leonard.* Yet, as I think of it now, black is a good contrast and so in fashion today.

"Excuse the smell. Fresh paint. They just redecorated the

hallway." I was leaning up against the door jamb. I quickly straightened up away from it, glancing at my elbow that had touched the wall.

He noticed. "It's okay. The paint's dry." A faint smile curved on his thin, pale lips. "Let's go down to my space."

Space?

He turned, opened another door off to the right behind the front door, and began descending a dimly lit stairwell.

About halfway down, the stairs turned left, and Leonard flipped a light switch on the wall. But no light came on. Then I saw the door at the bottom of the stairs, a slit of faint yellow light glowing at the bottom of it.

He reached the end of the stairs, turned the knob, and slowly opened the door.

We stepped into the room. A waft of warm, humid air blanketed my skin and stung my eyes. A pungent smell, similar to but fainter than skunk, hit my nostrils. I wanted to pull out my handkerchief and cover my nose. I relaxed and breathed shallowly.

I couldn't quite believe what I saw. There in the middle of the room were wire cages suspended from the ceiling by guywires at each corner of the cages. Inside the cages were squealing bats hanging from wood dowels placed at angles through the bars. There were varying numbers of bats per cage, from one to six. I recall there being about a half dozen cages. Very little bat guano was on the papers at the bottom of the cages. But what stool was there was watery and pale—not the normal pasty black of bat guano. The floor was linoleum over concrete. The concrete continued up at the sides to form half walls, with a shelf at about window level. The windows were painted black. From there to the high ceiling (eight or nine feet) was painted drywall.

I turned 360 degrees to get a clear picture of the room. It was then that I noticed our entrance had been through a double door with about four feet between the outside door and the inner one. At the other end of the room, twenty or so feet away, was another door, also a double door, "for security" as Leonard explained later. Off in corners of the room were garbage cans and a small refrigerator.

Leonard spoke. "This is my aviary. I open the cage doors and let them fly around for exercise."

"You do what?" I blurted out in surprise.

These were his "pets." And they got the best of care, he assured me. He cleaned the guano and washed walls of urine stain nightly. "Nightly," to him was any time he was awake and at home since, down here, there was no time, and daylight was artificial. He said he could "meld" with the bats; in response, they would wake up if asleep, and he would feed them and let them out to fly around the room.

He smiled and said, "I like to sit or lay here and listen to them flutter around, swooshing overhead. Free. Freeee," rolling the word around on his tongue, savoring it.

Free? But for cages and limited environment. And freedom for him to get rabies, I thought.

He went on to explain what the problem was that he called me about. It seems that, this past week, there was a sudden "epidemic" of diarrhea, starting with the bats at the back of the room and spreading forward. He thought some of them looked weak. He also wondered if maybe the nursing "moms" (of which there were two, each of which had one pup) were not producing enough milk for their young since the babies seemed more agitated and weak, one falling off the mother to the bottom of the cage. *Very unusual. What cave did he get them from that had a nursery so easily accessible that he could capture them?*

I shook my head in wonder at this strange nightmare unfolding before me. I sighed and proceeded with clinical thoughts out of habit. It was hard to believe what I was doing. Mixed feelings emerged: try to solve his problem versus the public health issue of rabies.

I asked several questions about changes in their environment, food, water, his comings and goings, if new utensils had been brought in, etc. He didn't know of any changes. He said his routine was the same and no new implements brought in. I asked him to detail a typical day. He said there was no "typical" day as far as when he came and went and when he opened the cages. Feeding was pretty much ad lib except that he liked to hand-feed several of them each time. *And get bitten?* I asked if he had a schedule as to which were handfed and in what order? No, he just started at the back of the room near the refrigerator where he kept the mealworms.

He fed both live and dried worms. Mealworms are actually not worms but insect larvae, immature stages of the darkling beetle. He would use forceps and present the live wiggly segmented worms one at a time to different bats—he seemed to distinguish ("know," as he said) each one from another. The dried worms he put in small dishes at the bottom of the cages, and the winged mammals would drop or climb to the bottom of the cage and crawl over and help themselves. Mealworms have an armor of chitinous segments, like the shells of shrimp. He said he loved to hear them crunching on the worms.

"It could get quite noisy with lots of them chomping down," he said.

Something was missing from his detail of history. Most of the time when there are stomach or intestinal problems, the root cause is something ingested. So I asked him more directly about the food items and source.

"Mr. Black, do you feed anything other than mealworms? Could the feed have gotten spoiled? How about fungus or some kind of discoloration among the worms?"

"Nope. My bats do well on them, and they like 'em. I keep 'em in the fridge. They don't look spoiled, do they?" And in a defensive tone of voice he added, "I always feed them fresh. I get new ones every week."

Puzzled, I decided it was time to look more closely at a few of the sick animals. I wasn't exactly afraid to touch them, but I was glad my rabies vaccination antibody titer was high. I asked him if he had a pair of supple leather gloves to handle the bats with. I didn't think they could bite through the leather. He didn't use gloves, he said, just his hands. I didn't like the idea of the sharp little needles stabbing into my fingers while I examined the critters. He offered to hold them while I looked. Reluctantly I said, "Okay." *Geez, I hope none of them are carrying rabies.*

We picked out the weakest-looking bats. He reached into the cage and grabbed the first one by the scruff of the neck. It flapped its wings in protest and twisted its head around trying to bite. Leonard took hold of the end of one wing and stretched it out so it wouldn't flap and get in the way of my inspection.

"The light is too dim." The ceiling lights were a string of yellow lightbulbs he had put together, purposely dim. "For their eyes. Bright light hurts their eyes," he explained.

I reached into my bag and pulled out a penlight and shone it on the first bat. "There, that's better."

His pets were all Mexican free-tailed bats, which are insectivores. Nearly half their length is in the tail—hence their name. This species of bat is the logo for the Bacardi rum company. It was chosen because they are beneficial to the sugarcane crops from which the rum is made. These bats eat the insect pests and pollinate the plants.

Under the first one's tail I could see some stool that was smeared around its anus. *No fresh red blood. Not pasty, more drippy. Not blacker than normal, as would be the case from bleeding in the digestive tract.* Stool color is sometimes black when there is bleeding higher up in the intestinal tract or in the stomach. Bats' guano is naturally dark because of their high-protein diet.

The mouth was easy to visualize since the little one squealed, its mouth open and its upper lip wrinkled, the whole time it was held. Nothing unusual there. I pinched the skin of its back. The "tent" I made with the pinch deflated slowly, indicating dehydration. I tried to palpate its internal organs by pushing a finger down on its abdomen. All I could feel was that there were some air bubbles mixed with the stool in the intestinal tract—a gaseous diarrhea, probably painful. Just then an impish side of me thought, *Mmm. Maybe some of the smell in the room is from multiple little farts.*

I examined one more, with similar results. Looking around in the cages, there was no fresh blood in any of the guano.

I washed my hands in the sink in the corner. "Bacteria-killing detergent," he assured me. *Just plain soap or detergent would have been better,* I thought.

I was mystified. *Something is missing.*

I opened the fridge to look through the batches of live meal-worms. They were in little plastic dishes, with pieces of oatmeal for food. Sifting through them, they looked okay to me. (*Though what would I know,* I thought. I don't see mealworms much, although I had used them once for fish bait.) There was the occasional brown-ish one. "Dead," Leonard explained. He said he discarded those, feeding only the healthy, pale yellow ones. There were a few others that were turning brown but appearing to shed their skin, molting. The dried ones were just that—dried up, desiccated.

I'm still missing something. I had a slew of questions. "You've been feeding the same things all along? No changes at all? When did your bats become ill? Did you change anything at all just before they came down sick? Are you sure you didn't bring in any new bats?"

"Yep, I'm sure. Only the moms are new, and they are in cages separate from the others. Nope, I've been feeding them the same."

"Is there anything different about your latest batch of food? Did you store them differently? Did you get new utensils? How about the water in the dishes in the cages? Was that any different?"

Something was not right. Something missing?

"I just use tap water," he said. I thought, *City water supply should be okay. Or did they change the chloride or fluoride in it or have a filtration error? Not likely.*

He cracked a smile again, swinging his gangly arms forward, animated. "The worms I get now are good and cheap."

"*Now?* What do you mean? Are some of the worms different?"

"Nope, the worms are the same. Good."

"You said 'now' and 'cheap.' Why are they cheaper?" I was getting animated myself. *Could this be the key? Are we onto something here?*

He elaborated, "I buy my worms from a guy who has cheaper ones. A friend at the bait shop told me about him. It costs me about half what I was paying before, and . . ."

I interrupted. "So now you get your worms from a different supplier. Now, you don't buy any from the previous source. Correct?"

"Yes, and . . ."

"When did you switch to the current batch of food?"

"About nine or ten days ago. I . . ."

My excitement peaked as I said, interrupting again, "And when did your pets begin getting sick? When did the diarrhea start?" My inner detective shouted, *Now we're getting somewhere!*

"I don't know. Mmm, maybe four or five days ago when . . ."

"Great. And did you switch over to the new worms immediately, or did you still have some of the former batch yet to feed them?"

"I only had a day's worth of the old stuff. I just get it when I need it, every week I . . ."

I couldn't contain myself, so I blurted out, "And you've bought from your new supplier a couple of times, and you ran out of the more expensive feed all at once and started feeding the cheap stuff all at once, with hardly any mix of old and new worms. Is that right?"

"Yes."

"Bingo!" I was putting it together. Finally. My inner epidemiologist was proud. At last I smiled. "Your new, cheaper food may not be so cheap after all."

He looked puzzled but not dumbfounded. A little agitated but not angry. "Do you think the new worms are poisoning my bats? I'm supposed to pick up some more worms from him tomorrow."

Trying to calm and reassure him, and maybe myself, too, I said, "No. No. Your bats are not being poisoned. Toxins in food act very quickly, within hours of feeding. For example, food poisoning, from staphylococcal toxins, in people usually starts within four to six hours after eating contaminated food."

"Whew, I guess they won't die then? They're not poisoned?"

"It's not poison, but I think the new food is making your bats sick. The incubation period, the time between first exposure and the onset of illness, was a few days, which is like that of an infection. An infection probably from a bacteria. Not a toxin."

"An infection? Bacteria? Do you mean I need to give antibiotics to my bats? How do I do that?" He whined, "My mealworms are clean; they don't look dirty. I clean my feeding cups and tweezers . . ."

"No, don't worry, you didn't contaminate the food. The worms probably had the bacteria inside them already, or it was a contamination of the oatmeal feed that came with them."

Trying to dissipate his angst, I said, "We don't know where the new supplier got the worms or what conditions he kept them in. All I'm saying is that the worms were already infected with the bacteria or virus before you got them."

He looked pensive, rocked back and forth. The tissue-paper skin of his face crinkled. A half smile. "Then the worms are sick, too."

"They are carrying the bacteria. But sometimes animals, and

even people for that matter, that carry disease-causing agents don't show any signs of illness themselves. Did you notice any more dead worms in the new batches compared to the previous ones?"

"Yep, there do seem to be more dark ones. I sort them out and discard them and only feed the yellow ones. But even throwing those away, these worms are still cheaper than the other bunch."

"Well, as I say, the healthy-looking ones can still carry the bacteria and make your bats sick." I smiled and added, "At least you don't have to give antibiotics to the mealworms!"

He sighed, not reacting to my attempt at levity. "What do I do about it, man? I need to buy more food tomorrow."

"The first thing you've got to do is not feed any more of the current batch of worms to your bats. We can get some canned baby food and . . ."

He cut me off (like I had cut him off before), shaking his head back and forth, "Baby food? Feed my bats baby food?"

"Well, yes." And with a chuckle, "The universal savior diet." Adding, "Just temporarily until you can get worms from your previous supplier—the more expensive but healthy worms. You can just put some baby food, almost any type, into dishes like you do your water, and your bats will crawl up to them and lap up the food." I didn't know if that was the case, but baby food works with other mammals. *It certainly works with cats and dogs.*

"Okay, I can get worms from my former guy in a day or so. What about antibiotics?"

I hesitated in answering. I had to admit that I was not familiar with what bacteria could be carried in mealworms, so I wasn't sure what antibiotic to use, if any. I did think of the possibility of salmonella bacteria, which are carried in a lot of wildlife and are a threat to humans. It also flashed through my mind that antibiotics often promote the "carrier" state, wherein the "bugs" go into hiding in the body for a period of time in a type of silent infection, only to be shed later and passed in stool to another animal or person.

I replied, "In order to determine which is the best antibiotic to use, ideally we should culture the stool and a few mealworms to find out which bacteria is there and to test that bacteria to see which antibiotic it's most susceptible to. But, Leonard, the culture and sensitivity testing takes time, and we can still do that if the diarrhea persists after changing the food.

"Let's get to your bats. I can give fluids to those I think are dehydrated." I saw the squint of worry on Leonard's brow and the raise of eyebrows in surprise, so I continued, smiling, "I don't need to put IV catheters in your bats and administer fluids with a drip. No, I'll just inject a small amount of the fluid under the skin, just what's needed to rehydrate. There will be a bump under the skin from the fluid, but it will go away quickly as the fluid is absorbed into the body."

He balked. "How much is all this going to cost? The fluids, the culturing of bacteria, the antibiotics. . ."

I gave him a verbal estimate of the costs of each item.

"Whew. Doc, I can't afford that. I don't have a job right now, and my parents don't want me . . ." A flush flashed briefly over his pale face. ". . . Well, I just can't handle it." Looking down and shaking his head, "My poor babies. My . . ."

I could feel his emotions sink, and I wasn't about to give him a spiel about the best care needed is blah, blah, blah.

"Look. Let's do what we can. You immediately stop feeding these worms. Buy some baby food, just for tonight and tomorrow morning until you can get the new worms from the former supplier. Throw out all the old worms—I'd have you feed them to the birds, but we don't want them to get sick too, do we?" I had no idea whether germs in mealworms could make a bird sick, but my comment seemed to make its point with Leonard.

He blushed again. Nodding, he said, "Okay. I get it. Flush down the toilet."

"Mmm, yeah. Clean out every cage and thoroughly wash anything that could be contaminated: the feed dishes, forceps, and water dishes. Rinse them in boiling water. Wash your hands between each cage or after handling anything that might be contaminated. Come to think of it, also get some yogurt to supplement, for just a couple of days, the new food you will get for them. The yogurt probiotic will introduce new, 'good,' bacteria into the bats' guts. You can do all that, right?" *Get him involved in the plan for cure.*

The blush on his face finally faded. "Sure, Doc, I can do that. I can do that."

I felt like I was on a roll but really only hoping my best guess would make things turn around quickly after getting off the bad batch of worms. "Great. And then after everything gets back to normal"—my fingers were crossed behind my back—"when the stools look solid, clean everything thoroughly again. Can you do that?"

"Yes. I'll do that, Doc. When do you think they'll get well?"

"Hopefully within one or two to four days."

"Awesome. I'll call the guy and get new mealworms today."

I hesitated but then decided I needed to let him know what I think and to warn him. "You know, Leonard, bats are wild animals. They need to live in the wild. Yours were caught outside and are captive." Thinking of his comment of being "free" to fly around the room, I added, "And they are not really *free*. Also, the most important part in my mind, there is the danger of rabies."

His dyed eyebrows rose. "You mean I could catch rabies? Isn't that hydrophobia? Like the mad dog in the movie *Cujo*?"

I continued, "I know you're careful in handling your bats, but the incubation period for rabies in bats is long, over a year in many cases and several years in some rare cases. So, it is possible your bats could be carrying the virus. I remember, Leonard, reading about a bat researcher who worked in a cave, not all that different from your basement here. The air in the cave was supersaturated with bat urine, and rabies virus can survive in bat urine for days. Anyway, the research doctor came down sick with rabies and died of the disease. He might have gotten it by inhaling the air in the cave that carried the virus or some of the urine mist may have gotten to him through a minor cut or skin wound." I winced, thinking *like the hangnail I have right now.* "Leonard, there is a lot of urine suspended in the air right here. I think . . ."

"But, I open these two windows and the back door and blow the air out with that fan." He pointed to a stand up fan in the back of the room. "I do it every few days. For the smell and also fresh air for my pets."

"That's all well and good, but I still highly—in fact, *urgently*—recommend you rethink your project here." Blinking, I said, "My eyes and nose are stinging from the humidity and the urine in this room."

Protesting, he said, "These are my pets. I love them."

What do I do with that? "I know. But consider that they were born free. Release them. Consider that they would have a vastly larger space to fly in than in the limited confines of your basement. Consider that you would be safer, and your bats would not get sick from contaminated mealworms. They would have more natural feed, insects they could catch on the wing. And they would be *free*! *Freee*"—drawing out the word—"to . . ." From the sudden crinkling of his forehead, I could see that the lightbulb went on in his head.

"Yes, I . . ." Silence, nodding his head. *Was that a tear in the corner of his eye?*

"Think about what I've said. Remember to wash your hands frequently. Get yourself some gloves." I reached into my bag and pulled out a package of latex exam gloves. "Here, you can have these. Bat saliva, the most common source of rabies virus in California, can get into minor cuts on your fingers that you don't even notice. So wear these when handling them. Let's go upstairs and finish our discussion there." I was beginning to feel suffocated by the heavy air and thinking about the guy who died inhaling the cloud of bat urine.

We went out through the double doors and ascended the staircase. He switched out the lights below.

As I stepped out into the hall, my eyes squinted. The brilliant sun shone through the front door, still open. I smiled at the splash of color in the rug. I inhaled a deep breath of fresh air.

Gathering myself to deliver more bad news, I said, "Leonard, there is another problem. The state of California requires people who keep wild animals captive to apply for a permit that is issued by the Department of Fish and Game. And I know they will not give you a permit to house bats. Bats are a 'restricted' animal in California."

He stood there, not saying a thing. He had a look of what I interpreted as disbelief on his face. I let him turn that over in his mind.

"Wait here. I'm going to take my bag to the car and make out the bill. I'll be right back."

When I returned, it struck me again how pale he was and the contrast of his black clothes to the bright hallway. His mouth was downturned. Then he said, "I don't have a permit. What'll I do? My babies."

"Leonard, I'm not a policeman. I won't report you. But please do the right thing. Let your pets go free. Don't risk catching rabies. It's fatal."

He stood there, clearly thinking about what I said. "I could apply to the state for a permit. Who?"

I shook my head. "You could. But, as I said, it won't be granted. It's too dangerous."

"Okay, what do I owe you?"

I handed him a copy of the bill.

He asked me to wait. He had to go down the hall to Mom's room. "She keeps money there for me." He returned, cash in hand, saying, "Thank you. I really do thank you for coming."

"And thank you, Leonard. Please think about what I said. Freedom, freeeedom. Release them from confinement. Give me a call in a day or two and let me know how things are going, if the diarrhea episode is ended." Pausing. "If it continues, maybe there is something else we can do to make sure they are healthy when you release them. But most of all, their freeeedom."

He nodded. "It's okay. I'll take care of it."

As I walked out the sidewalk toward my car, I turned around and saw him standing back a little, near the door to the basement. I shouted, "And be sure to get plenty of *fresh* air," waving my hands in a wide arc above me.

As I turned and walked the next few steps to my car, I heard him call out while closing his door, "I do. Every night."

I did hear again from Mr. Black. He was elated. He said everything was back to normal. No diarrhea, and the bats were strong enough to have no trouble flying around now. When I asked about him and how he was managing the new, careful routine, he said, "Great." He told me that he'd thought about what I said and added that he was freeing his beloved insectivores. I was delighted to hear that and told him so.

Then he added, "And I think I'll get some fruit-eating bats, flying foxes. I think fruit will be easier than worms. Besides, I like their scientific name. *Pteropus vampyrus.*"

12

Ratty Yes, Batty No

I first met Ms. June Jewel when she presented her sick rat, Candy, for examination at a veterinary hospital. I was filling in for a doctor who was temporarily away, attending a veterinary conference for continuing education. Candy was a brown-and-white Norway rat, weighing about three quarters of a pound. She was cute but also cuddly, for which I was most grateful as she didn't try to bite me. Handling rats does not always come nip-free.

Candy had an abscess on one of her rear legs (a "love" bite from her mate) which I drained and flushed with disinfectant. She didn't struggle, not even when I gave her an antibiotic injection. *Wish all my exotic patients were that cooperative!*

When I handed Candy back to Ms. Jewel, she enfolded her pet rat into a towel and said, "Oh, please call me June." We struck up a conversation. She heard I did house calls and asked for my phone number. The receptionist at the front desk gave her my business card.

She later called to have me come over to her "shop" to see her other pet rats.

The neighborhood was an old part of Orangevale, wood-frame houses built after World War II. The house she lived in was typical, small, a little overgrown in hedges in the front, with an uneven walkway. Some sections of the concrete were cracked and upheaved by roots of a large oak tree. It was summer and the crabgrass was yellowing and creeping over the edges of the sidewalk.

I drove in and parked in the long driveway on the side of her house. The day had been in triple-digit temperatures, common for summer in the Sacramento Valley, and I was tired after a long day. This was my last call. I stepped out of my comfortable air-conditioned car and into the valley air, like stepping into a blast furnace. Walking up the driveway, carrying my medical satchel, I took only a few steps, and the sweat began to drip.

June was waiting in front of the garage, sitting in a fold-up web chair that seemed to wrap around her tiny frame. She wore her graying reddish hair tied into a bun at the back of her head. Six-tyish, tanned, still freckled. She wore a light blue T-shirt with "I ♥ rats" on it, khaki shorts, and faded gray tennis shoes, sans socks. She stood and waved as I trudged up the seemingly endless, steamy pavement. Her smile was broad.

The sight brightened my outlook, and I did look forward to seeing her rats. She said they were her "business."

We shook hands in friendly greeting. "Did you find the house easily?" Then came the savior question, "Would you like some iced tea?"

"June, yes, and yes, I sure would like some iced tea," I said, wiping a finger like a squeegee across my wet brow.

"Well, good. I'll run inside and get us both a cold one." She turned and ascended the back porch with a youthful spring in her steps, calling back, "I'll just be a minute," and disappeared into the house. *A minute might be too long. A real "cold one"—a brew—would be nice.*

After she returned with the iced tea, we exchanged a few niceties and commented on the weatherman's predictions of a continuing hot spell. Then she got down to business, telling me how her rats were her livelihood and her pets. She pushed a button on a remote in her hand. The gray door in the detached, white, wood-framed garage rose. There they were, all hundred-plus adults and their litters.

Wire cages were stacked one on top of another in three vertical towers, unlike Mr. Black's horizontal rows of cages. Each cage had a pullout metal bottom tray with a floor lining of wood shavings or other fibrous material. There was a large washing tub in the middle of the garage, with a garden hose strung out from the tub through a hole in the garage wall, presumably connected to a spigot out back. The air had a somewhat pungent smell, like Pine-Sol. Next to the tub were pans and water bottles leaning against each other, draining onto the cement floor, which had a groove running through the floor to the back of the garage to a drain hole, covered with tight screen mesh. She had scrub brushes and other implements hanging on hooks from the ceiling. I stepped into her cave of rats, the cages on each side of me like stalagmites.

Then I felt it. A flow of cool air brushing my face. A welcome breeze indeed. I asked about it.

She pointed to a swamp cooler mounted up high on a side wall, a window cutout, and wood braces supporting the cooler. "Oh." I inhaled the coolness. "It's so quiet and efficient. How did you get a swamp cooler that quiet?"

"At a garage sale last year. Works good, doesn't it?" Smiling, with pride. "Guess I just got lucky."

Time to turn our attention to business, I thought. "Well, June, what's been happening? How are your rats? What is the business?"

June grinned, "I raise a lot of rats for pet stores. So others can enjoy them as I do. I get a good price, especially for the cute little ones."

"So you have your own stock of breeding pairs . . ."

"All you got to do, Doc, is put two of the right ones together, and 'pow' you've got babies," she said, snapping her fingers. "Doesn't take much after that to raise them to weaning, when I can sell 'em to the pet stores. Only problem is that sometimes I get attached to one of them, like Candy, and can't let her go."

Her face changed from a grin to a serious business look. "Then there are the others. The ones I raise not to breed but for individual buyers. Food. For their snakes."

Pets . . . and food for other pets! The incongruity struck me. Pets as food was ironic enough to me. I wasn't sure how I felt. Mother Nature has her ways. *She does seem to love her rats.*

Shaking my head to recover the present moment, I swept my hand in the air in a swishing arc around the room. "Quite an operation, June. What can I do for you today?" I observed that there were some husbandry changes that could be made to improve the standard of care. But also, it was clear to me that she was really trying to do a good job.

"I've got a couple of sneezing ones and a charming momma that refuses to be a momma. Then there is Sami. He's my oldest and best breeder, and he has a large lump near his leg. Poor dear just drags it along with him. Doesn't stop him mating," she giggled, "and the girls don't seem to mind it. Doctor MacVean, I'd like you to take a look at everything and tell me what I can do better."

Good attitude. Real problems. "Let's just take a walk around your garage. You point out your concerns when we come to them, and I'll point out mine."

"Okay. Sounds good. Where do you want to start?"

"Let's start right where we are. When you clean cages or change water bottles, or just open a cage for whatever reason, how do you keep one of them from slipping out and escaping into the neighborhood?" I could see that the door at the rear, presumably leading to the backyard, did not go all the way to the floor. With only an inch and a half or so of space, a rat could easily squeeze its way out. Also, there were only two tiny lightbulbs strung across the ceiling for lighting. "Do you keep the garage door open for lighting when you work in here? And I'm concerned . . ."

"In good weather, like now"—*What good weather?*—"I do keep it open—except when there are too many nosy people walking by. In the winter, I keep it closed. Gets cold, and the winds rush through, whipping things into a mess sometimes. Too much cleaning up. It really helped, me getting the automatic door opener. Only problem is that I keep losing the darn remote. And sometimes it's because I'm carrying it in my pocket!"

"Ha, that's good. I know that one." I shared with her that I don't lose the garage door opener since it is stationed on the windshield visor of my car. "But, boy, is it frustrating those times I lose my TV remote. Especially in the fall and winter, when I want to watch my beloved football. I have withdrawal symptoms when I can't watch a game on the weekend. I get really peeved when I can't constantly change channels to watch several games at once because I've lost my remote!"

She laughed and said, "My ex-husband used to hog the TV all weekend. College football on Saturday and professional football on Sunday. He changed channels back and forth all the time. It drove me nuts. I fixed the problem. I kept the remote and got rid of him!"

I chuckled. "Well, I gotta admit, he sounds a little like me during football season."

Getting back to the rat escape issue, I pointed out how one could get through the bottom of the back door and how that could easily be remedied by fixing a weather strip there. She got the clipboard that was hanging on a wall with a pencil attached by a string. She began a "To Do" list.

"Okay, what next?" she asked.

I didn't think we'd fully addressed the question of escape of rats into the neighborhood, so I asked the question again.

"Some of those little buggers are escape artists. Now I keep the garage door down when I know I'm going to be opening the cage of those little rascals. But sometimes they get out. Most I'm able to catch with my fishnet." She pointed her sparrow-thin fingers toward a long-handled net that hung on a wall.

She continued, "Occasionally, one is lost. Maybe getting out under the door like you pointed out. I only had one, Shirley, who got out by way of the garage door. I hadn't shut it all the way. Darn, and she was pregnant at the time."

My mind jumped to a picture of Shirley holing up in a neighbor's wall or something and a whole bunch of little rats becoming residents of the neighborhood. "Did you capture her? What do the neighbors think?"

Sadness washed over her face. Shaking her head, "No. I never got her back." *Was that a tear welling up in her eye?* "I couldn't bear going around the neighborhood asking if they had seen my Shirley. They think I'm batty as it is. Well, not all of them. Some see it as a business, but they did ask about zoning rules. They don't know how much I love my pets. And I never let my cats in here."

"Sorry you couldn't prevent Shirley from escaping," I said, shaking my head. I genuinely felt sorry myself, just seeing her so upset and the loss on her face. Even rats rate love. "But we can do something about it. To fix your place so no others can escape." The conditions here were not ideal, and there was no way to keep her garage escape-proof. I told her about a book by A. L. Williams I once read that had a title that told it all: *All You Can Do Is All You Can Do But All You Can Do Is Enough!*

The sunshine came out from behind the cloud. "Oh, yes. Of course. The weather stripping. And I suppose sealing any cracks around hoses and piping and seams?" Answering her own question, "Yes. And I already put wire mesh at the drain."

I smiled back and got my professional face back on. "Another concern of mine is that there is a lot of crowding in here." It was just a one-car garage—the norm back when her house was built. "The aisles between the cages are narrow, so not much room for you to do your work. I know you want to do maintenance cleaning and feeding, changing water bottles, and all the things you need to do. But with such narrow aisles, it's not easy, and it would be possible for you to lose another of your 'pets.'"

"So we need to figure out a way to widen the aisles. Mmmm . . ." she said, rubbing her chin. "I might be able to move the cleaning tub outside into the back. Mmmm, maybe do something different to store the utensils and feed bins . . ." Her mind was whirring.

"I'm sure you'll figure out a way. Let's mosey on down the rows and see what we can see." I stepped between the row of cages against the left wall and one of the middle rows. Looking up and down, peering into cages, it was clear she really kept after cleaning. But there was a problem. "June, you've done a good job stacking the cages . . ."

"Oh, thank you, I . . ."

"But they are stacked too high for the conditions you have here."

"What do you mean?" Puzzled.

"Look how the sawdust shavings from the top cages spill out the side onto the cages below. If there is a contagious illness, like a respiratory problem, like your sneezing ones"—a common issue with rats—"and the discharges that cling to the shavings spills over onto the bottom cages, the disease could be spread to the others below." She began to frown. "Get my point?"

Scratching the bun on top of her head, "I'm not sure. I stacked them pretty carefully."

"I know you have." Pointing out one of the top cages that sat back a little, I brushed some of the shavings over the edge, letting it spill onto the cage below. And brushing a little harder, like a rat might manage to do when shuffling space to sleep or build a nest in a corner.

"Oh, I see." She paused and scratched the bun again, a concerned look on her face. "Yes, sometimes I spill stuff myself when I am on my ladder to take care of the top cage." The cages were stacked three high, with the bottom ones resting on low benches. "What do you think I can do about it? I don't want stuff like snot spilling down to others."

"Yes, like snot," I said, smiling inside. "Well, the best thing in my opinion is to reduce the rows to one cage high."

An objection formed on her expressive face.

"Ah, ah, I know, that really cuts into your bottom line."

She shook her head.

I continued, "Maybe you could build shelves between the stacks and just extend the shelves out a little beyond the cages to catch the spillovers."

Nodding, she said, "That I could do, but then they'd be even higher. I'd have to get a taller ladder." Her voice trembling just a bit, she added, "And I'm not as steady as I used to be, so the ladder business might be risky."

"I imagine it's risky now." I smiled, trying to keep the exchange light.

A flash of thought, eyebrows lifting, "Maybe I could lower the legs on the benches, so the first level is lower, and the highest cage wouldn't be so high. Then maybe I could simply use the ladder I have."

"I'm sure you'll figure out a way. But I think you should make a whole lot more room for yourself and your rats by reducing to fewer cages—to correct the height and the aisle spacing problems. I know fewer cages . . ."

Interjecting, "You know . . ." she paused. "I've been thinking of building on to the back of the garage. Maybe extending the wall so I would have more space. Of course, I was thinking of more cages. But from what you've said, maybe I'll do it but with only the cages I already have." A sneaky smile curled at the edge of her mouth, "And maybe just a *few* more cages."

I chuckled. "Uh huh, just a *few* more," I said, shaking my head. That made her laugh. It felt good. I finished with my comments regarding husbandry of her colony and asked after the sick ones.

Nodding her head, she said, "The sniveling ones are getting better now. And, as you said, I can stop it spreading to others by keeping the shavings from being shared." Then she added, "But I do have one female who won't get pregnant, and then there's Sami. He's over there in the back."

We walked over to his cage. Looking in, I saw a small, gray-ish-brown Norway male with a huge mass in his groin area that was nearly a third the size of his body. I reached in and, holding Sami by the scruff of the neck, palpated the growth. He had both testicles, and the mass was not attached to either. In fact, it was loose under the skin. Just HUGE. I released him and watched as he shuffled along the bottom of the cage, dragging his baggage along with no trouble at all. "It doesn't seem to bother him much, does it?"

"No, sir, he seems to get along just fine. And, as I said, the girls don't seem to mind it." And with a childish giggle, "They just think he has more balls than the others!"

Smiling but with a serious tone of voice, I said, "It's probably a benign tumor, not cancer. I can't really say until I take a sample of the tissue, which I can do with a needle and syringe. But that's rather academic if you are going to have it removed anyway. And that is what I would recommend since, look there." I pointed to a reddened area of the skin below the tumor. "See where the redness is? He may soon develop an ulcer and infection there where he is dragging it along the bottom of his cage. And it could eventually grow to a size where it impedes his movements and maybe presses on some veins, blocking blood flow."

She asked about the cost of doing it, and I explained what would be involved with antisepsis, anesthesia, antibiotics, surgical proce-dure, and quoted her a price. I let her know I couldn't do it right then because it was the end of a long day for me. I was beat. "But we could find a time and day that would work for both of us next week. And I can also evaluate that little cutie that doesn't want to be a momma."

She thought a while. "Okay. Let's do it. Sami is one of my best breeders." And with a wide grin, added, "How long do you think it'll keep him 'out of operation?'"

"Gosh, June, as tough as Sami looks, I suspect he will be back at it in no time. The stitches will be buried, under the skin, so they won't tickle his girlfriends!"

I had the pleasure of seeing June on subsequent house calls. Besides consulting with her on her business, I was referred to several of her customers—reptile lovers who bought her rats for food, for their scaled pets, of course.

13

Freddy and Friends

By early winter when temperatures had fallen, several of June's referrals called. One of them was John Coluber. He was tall, slender, and active. His moves were smooth, such that he seemed to just glide across the floor when he walked—a sort of reverse moonwalk. He lived in one of the classic Victorian houses, so common in midtown Sacramento, which had been converted to apartments. He rode his mountain bike or ran miles every morning. He left his top-floor apartment before breakfast, usually taking the trails along the American River to where it joins the Sacramento River and then continued his run through the tourist area of Old Sacramento and was back by the time most people begin breakfast. He said he'd be so endorphin-high that he'd forget to eat and simply rode his bike directly to work at the post office, where he sorted mail and did "whatever," as he put it.

John called regarding his green iguana. "Skinny" was not himself of late. All eighteen inches of body plus about thirty inches of tail (nearly two thirds of his length!) stretched out on the bottom of his cage, legs splayed. He was barely able to get to his water dish and wouldn't eat like usual. He was losing weight.

"In fact, he has lost so much weight my roommate has gone to calling him 'skinny Skinny.' His ribs always used to show, but not this much."

John led me to the large dining area, which was dark except for a small incandescent lightbulb over Skinny's cage. The table on which the cage rested was up against the far wall. *Interesting! To place an iguana cage on the end of the dining table? Oh well, there is plenty of room on the dinner table.* I also began to imagine what dinner conversations were like when guests were over.

The cage certainly was big enough. There were a couple of climbing branches. But the iguana just hovered in one corner of the cage with a drawn look on its face. *Imagine a drawn-faced lizard.*

Skinny's skin color was more gray than green. Of course, I couldn't quite trust that assessment. I am partially green and red colorblind, just enough so I can't distinguish between light green and gray. Not letting a little thing like that deter me, I informed John that his iguana's color was "fading," a common occurrence as iguanas age. But, Skinny was a young five-year-old. I informed John that if we can solve the problem Skinny might live another fifteen years or more. That's not uncommon in captive iguanas. In the wild they only reach about ten to fifteen years.

I cautiously leaned over the cage to pick up Skinny. Caution is always the word with handling iguanas because of their sharp rows of teeth, sixty to a hundred of them, which are continually replaced with more teeth behind as the jaw lengthens, kinda like the continuous regeneration of the teeth of sharks. And their claws are like daggers. I slipped one hand under his belly and the fingers of my other hand around the tail. If the tail is not restrained, one can get a nasty whiplash across the face. I got smacked by one of the tails of a patient, and it hurt worse than I imagined an insulted woman's slap across the face would feel like.

Skinny didn't seem to mind being lifted, and I felt bumps along the bones of his spine. When I started to push fingers in on his belly to attempt to palpate his innards, he struggled as if in pain and tried to bite. I quickly put him down. Instead of attempting to scamper away, he just lay there, panting. Unusual behavior for an iguana.

I had gotten a quick feel of his ribs. They weren't solid, more rubbery. I looked at his gaping mouth with the teeth. *I think I'd best not handle him anymore right now*, my defensive thoughts trying to justify not probing more into scratching-biting territory just yet. *Look at his environment instead, the most likely issue anyway.*

I noticed another cage. It was much larger than Skinny's cage and hung over the edges of a table on the side wall opposite the door to the kitchen. "Do you transfer Skinny to the other cage sometimes?"

Chuckling, "Oh, no, that's for Freddy. He's not feeling so hot himself, so while you're here I want you to take a look at him, too."

The thermometer at the back of Skinny's cage read slightly above current room temperature, 72°F. *Too cool for a tropical animal. They don't possess a temperature regulation system. Plenty of greens in the cage for Skinny to eat. Looks like a cricket darting under that leaf. I wonder about a cricket in a vegetarian's diet.* I smiled at the idea of the protein supplement.

"John, the lightbulb is too high above the cage to give much heat. Do you set the cage out in the sunlight at all? Your balcony is south-facing and must get plenty of natural light."

"Nah, I didn't think it was a good idea to expose him to the automobile fumes from the street below. But I do let him out into the dining and living rooms. Well, I used to, before he got sick."

"John, I think Skinny has metabolic bone disease, a common problem for iguanas. He is not getting ultraviolet light, which he needs for absorbing calcium into his body and into his bones. As a consequence his bones are thin. I believe he may even have multiple fractures as a result. Enough to make it too painful to move. Also, with this disease his jaw is rubbery and maybe even fractured, so that he can't chew properly."

"Rubbery jaws? He needs light?"

"Yes, specifically ultraviolet, UV, light. Which is provided by natural sunlight, or you can buy a UV lamp or one of the new 'natural light' bulbs to place over Skinny's cage."

"UV lamp? Uhh." He was mulling that idea over in his head. Then, as if the lightbulb in his brain lit up, he said, "Oh, you mean like what my roommate has over the plants in his closet?" And, in a seemingly joking tone of voice, John added, "Say, you're not a cop, are you?"

Smiling, thinking *You're not the first to question that,* I answered, "John, I'm not a cop."

He cocked his head and lifted an eyebrow, thinking about it a bit. Then he motioned for me to follow him. He led me to a darkened bedroom way in the back of the apartment. We walked past a pile of clothes and papers to a closet on the side of the room. I noticed in passing through that shirts, belts, and a pillowcase were hung on chairs and loose on the bed. *A bachelor pad for sure. And what does that cage in the corner on the other side of his roommate's bedroom hold?*

He opened the closet door, and I was practically blinded and had to lift my arm to shield my eyes from the light.

"Are these the kind of lamps you mean?"

My eyes adjusted. Two rows of potted pot plants reached up toward a row of three very bright UV lamps. "Yup. That's them. That's what you need. Your roommate uses them for greening his weed. You need to use one to green yer iguana."

He squinted, raised his eyebrows, and said, "You're not going to report this are you? Sal is just growing it for his own use. He doesn't sell his pot. Just for himself. Well, sometimes I take a toke."

"As maybe a few of his close friends do," I added. "No, John, I'm not a policeman, and I don't report things that are none of my business."

An audible, "Whew."

"I don't believe it should be illegal anyway," I said, smiling and turning away from the sunlamps.

Walking out of the room, I asked what was kept in Sal's cage. He told me it was his roommate's snake, Boo. Having noticed the cage was empty, I wondered *And where is Boo? Lots of hiding places in that room.*

We walked back over to Skinny's cage, and I showed him where to place the UV bulb over the cage, not too high so it would provide enough light and give off heat, but not so low that it would be too hot for him. "He needs heat as well. Iguanas, as I know you know, live in nature in the tropics. So, Skinny needs heat on the order of seventy-eight to ninety-two degrees. And, John, fix up your balcony with a cage to keep him in, so he can bask in the sun. Put him out in that cage every day the weather is conducive. Lots of sunlight, natural light."

"Okay, I got it. Get better light for him. When do you think he'll be better?"

"Real soon. In a matter of two or three weeks he will be moving better. And we can increase the calcium in his diet." I gave him a handout on methods of force-feeding if needed and ways of slipping calcium to him. I told him about how in tropical countries I'd seen pet iguanas tethered to stakes in their caretaker's yards, a leash around the neck, so the lizard could bask in the sun and not escape.

"Say, what about Freddy? Do you think he needs sunlight also?"

"Who's Freddy? Oh yes, the one from the cage next to the kitchen?"

John held up his hand, moved me to the edge of his living room and told me to stay there. He hustled in his reverse moonwalk way into the kitchen, grabbed an object out of the refrigerator, and returned to stand beside me. He threw the object out onto the middle of the wood floor. Plop! Almost immediately a very large lizard darted out from under the sofa to my right and grabbed the object, a rat. I almost stumbled backward at the surprise and suddenness of the attack.

Recovering my bearings, I looked at the dark twenty-four-, maybe thirty-inch-long creature with shiny bead-like scales and said, "Ah, a monitor lizard." *Related to the Komodo Dragon!*

With glee, he swung his arms in an arc and said, "Yep, a monitor. Hee, hee. I love doing that when I have guests over who haven't seen this before. Sometimes Fred will dash out right between their legs and scare the bejeezus out of 'em! Ha, one girl jumped up onto the couch screaming like she'd seen a mouse. Of course she sort of had—a rat, anyway." He went on to explain that he usually pitched a live rat, and that Freddy would scurry and grab it before it took two steps. He added, "But I didn't have a live one today, only that frozen one. He'll eat it, even stone cold. Actually, he is so friendly I can pick him up and cuddle him. I'll kiss him on the cheek, and he'll lick my ear with his long forked tongue. My girlfriend and I will be on the living room couch watching TV and Freddy will be snuggling in between us."

He's a little odd, I thought, *somewhat like Mr. Leonard Black.*

Settling down some from his excitement, John said, "Hey, do you think Freddy would benefit from that sunlight and UV? He's been kind of sluggish lately. Ha, I know you wouldn't know it from how fast he moved just now. But he must have been pretty hungry to move that fast. He hasn't been eating well lately. Hey, Doc, while you're here"—*Oh, I've heard that a million times*—"could you take a look at Freddy?" *It's not really a question.* "Maybe he is sick." *Okay, I tell myself, but I've got to remember to add a second pet physical exam to the bill.*

John scurried over and took the rat out of Freddy's mouth and pinned him to the floor—neck in one hand and tail in the other. I went over, kneeled down, and looked him over. Then I took a penlight out of my shirt pocket and looked at the eyes, lids, lips. I prodded the mouth open with the penlight and peered in as best I could. All looked normal.

"So far, so good." Then I palpated his sides, first the ribs and chest, then slid my fingers along the sides and under the belly, feeling as deep as I could. *Ah, what's this?*

"Okay, John, I need you to lift him up when I tell you to." Then I went over and retrieved a Q-tip swab from my bag and a tube of lubricant and lubricated the end of the swab. "All right, now turn him over slowly, belly up." I then pushed the Q-tip into the anus, the natural slit-like opening in the belly at the end of the abdomen and midway between the hind legs. "Now you can turn him back over and release him to finish the meal."

I smiled, shaking my head. He said, "What. What's wrong? What did you find?"

"I have news for you, John. Freddy is actually Frederica."

"What do you mean, Frederica?"

"Well, *he* is a *she*."

"But the store clerk said he was 'Fred.'"

"Yes, but he also didn't tell you the need for light and warmth for Skinny, did he?"

I went on to explain that the slit in the belly is the opening to a bag-like chamber called the cloaca, the common receptacle through which passes excrement, urine, and reproduction. "In your monitor the Q-tip went into the cloaca too far to be a male. That's because there is no penis in your monitor. Since a monitor's penis is fluke-like, coiled up like a spring, filling the cloaca, the Q-tip can only go a very short way in a male."

"Whoa, man, so she's a girl?"

"Yep. Also, I felt a soft lump inside the belly, which could be an egg developing. They don't need a male around to lay. Of course the egg would not be fertile. Usually when the female lizard goes into a laying cycle she loses her appetite and becomes somewhat lethargic. Anyway, John, that might explain what's going on with her."

"Wow. That's too much. Way cool. Will she be okay now?"

"Likely. But if she has trouble passing the egg, a condition we call 'egg-bound,' or if she gets much more lethargic and doesn't eat at all, give me a call." Peering past John I saw that Frederica was chowing down on the frozen meal. "I think she'll be all right."

"Gee, thanks. 'Frederica!' Ha, I like it. Hey, man, while you are here . . . could you look at Boo? He, or she . . ."

Interrupting, I glanced at my watch. "No, I'm afraid not. I have another house call to make today, and it's getting late. Another time." Pulling my receipt slips out of my bag, I added, "I'll just total up the bill." I finished and handed the bill to him, which included the *two* physicals. He paid in cash, something I always appreciate. "Gotta go." *It has been an interesting call to say the least.*

Then I heard it. *CRUNCH.* The frozen rat was snapped in two by the monitor's bite.

John exclaimed, "Ha. It looks like 'Frederica's' jaws are not rubbery!"

14

Monster at the End of the Hall

I turned the corner into a long hallway. A dim light glowed through a door which was ajar at the other end of the hall. There, in the middle of the corridor, limned by the silhouetting light, loomed the round dark hulk of the creature. It looked huge, coming up to my mid-thigh and as wide as it was tall. In the dark hallway I couldn't tell how long it was, and the odd light of the gloom stretched it out in my mind like a locomotive.

Perhaps I'd guessed its weight too low. Did I have enough sedative to do the job? I fingered the hypodermic syringe and attached needle in my right hand, felt along the edge of the rug with my shoe, steadying myself with my left hand along the smooth wood-paneled wall. I couldn't make out its head, just a round black formlessness. I needed to inject a muscle, preferably into its thigh; but anywhere in its haunches would do. I needed to get deep into a muscle. If I injected into fat, tissue with little blood supply to absorb the drug, it would take forever for the sedative to do its work.

I slowly inched my way along, fully expecting it to run farther down and into the room at the end of the hall.

Then, I saw the white glistening of its eyeballs. It was looking right at me. With a sudden explosion of energy, it launched itself straight for me! A swiftness of bulk that knocked me over like a bowling pin. I fell forward, feet out from under me, onto its back. It was carrying me ass-backward down the hall, clomping and squealing like the whistle of a full-bore locomotive charging toward the living room. The tail was flapping in front of my face, so I grabbed it at its base and held on tight. I bounced as if in a bone-jarring rodeo, the beast's ridge of a backbone jabbing into my chest and belly.

I gathered my wits quickly enough against the shock of the attack to raise my right hand and plunge the hypo into the curve of body to the left of his tail. Just then the bull monster jerked left and the needle, a hefty 19-gauger, bent to nearly a 90-degree angle in its tough hide.

Glancing at the syringe, I figured I could still get what was left of the fluid through the needle if I could get it through the skin. I plunged again, this time striking a thinner portion of hide just below and to the side of the tail. The plunger pushed all the way, but I had no idea if there was enough sedative left to do the job.

And the bristly ride had just begun.

My legs flailing out behind me and a hard ridge of a backbone digging into my gut and a painful blow into my groin, I tried to fall off. But just as I managed to lean to one side and was about to fall, the bounding bull would lunge in the direction I was falling so that I bounced back up onto the ridge. This bouncing, leaning, and bucking back and forth continued for what seemed like forever. Enough to knock the wind out of me.

Worse, I worried about the crashing of furniture and glass as we bounded around the rodeo ring, formerly called a living room. I feared it would look like the swath of a tornado. When I finally did fall off, my back hit something solid, glass rattled, and objects broke.

I glanced up and saw it turn back toward me. But it had slowed and was weaving in a drunken path. The sedative seemed to be kicking in. *Could some of it have gotten injected directly into the bloodstream? Thank goodness*, I sighed. *Taking effect quickly.* I certainly didn't have the time or steadiness to pull back the plunger to see blood flow up into the syringe, which would indicate I was in a vein. If in a vein, it might be too heavy of a dose, assuming there was enough fluid still left in the hypo. And it wouldn't keep the beast sedated as long as if in muscle.

Rolling out of the way and onto my feet, staggering, trying to get my wind back, I dizzily surveyed the battlefield. Not as bad as I thought. Then my eyes focused. Lots of items had been knocked over, but no apparent breakages. *Oops, the china closet against the wall.* Pieces of glass figurines and pottery littered the shelves.

Stepping off to the side, I apologized to Mr. and Mrs. Calmer for all the mess—especially the china items, not to mention the knickknacks strewn about the room and knocked over end tables.

The couple had such matter-of-fact expressions on their round faces. They assured me that it was okay and that they were used to it.

I wondered how they could be so relaxed about it.

Mr. Calmer stroked his soft short white beard with one hand while the other rested on his ample belly, explaining, "Don't pay no mind. Anything valuable we leave out of the living room." He added that they don't put "good stuff" anywhere their potbellied pig, Charley, might cruise.

Mrs. Calmer, hands across her midriff, nodding, continued almost with the same breath where hubby left off. "Charley is wont to bull his way around the house on occasion."

Mr. followed as if continuing his wife's sentence with, "Sometimes he's just letting us know he's hungry."

In tandem, Mrs. added, "Sometimes he does it to let us know he wants to go outside and root in the garden." She curled her lips and said, "I purposefully don't let him out into my precious garden. But Charley knows how to get even—by pushing something over with his snout or rooting up a throw rug."

On cue, as if in a relay, Mr. laughed. "But other times he does it just for fun!"

It wasn't really so bad, they assured me. His antics often gave them a good laugh, especially when they played "go fetch the paper." Mr. said, "I roll up the newspaper and wrap it with a rubber band so it keeps its shape and is easy to pick up."

Mrs. added, "And one of us tosses it about in the backyard." Mrs. laughed. "It's funny to see him fetch it and then stand panting afterward waiting for the next throw, just like a dog."

Looking back and forth between each other, they chorused, "We're not sure if pigs can swim, so we never toss the paper stick into the pool."

I assured them, "Actually, pigs can swim quite well."

Mr. tapped his belly and ribs while replying, "Ha, he'd probably float like I do, having so much 'meat' on his bones."

Mrs. chimed in, "He likes it when we add water to his mud hole in the corner of the yard." She swished her hands in front of her.

"Ha, yes, they don't sweat like we do," I chimed in, "so they love wallowing in mud to cool off. Charley would probably like a dip in the pool on a hot summer day. But make sure you have good steps or a rough-surfaced nonslip ramp so he can get in and out of your pool easily."

"Yep," Mr. replied, "he would have a hard time getting out of our pool."

"And we made sure he can't get in it, either," added Mrs. with a smile, "'cause we built a fence around it." Turning toward her husband, hands on hips, she said, "And when are you going to build a fence around my garden?"

Meanwhile, enough of the sedative had gotten into Charley's system so that he stopped romping around the room and squealing at the top of his lungs. When he stopped and stood as if in a stupor,

I attempted to push him over onto his side so I could begin the veterinary procedures.

Feeling my push against his skin, he just snorted and galloped forward a few paces. *Well, guess I'll just have to add to the drug cocktail.*

As I filled a second syringe, I explained to the Calmers that I would inject another dose, but on the low dose side, for safety. *And just what dose do you guess will do the trick? You don't know how much you actually got into him and how much is still lingering in the muscles slowly dumping into his bloodstream.* I figured he might have been over two hundred pounds. My mind further injected self-doubt— *You've never dealt with a pig this big since veterinary school, and even then not with an injectable anesthetic or sedative.* But "Challenge" is my middle name, so I went with my best educated guess.

Now, if he will just stay still long enough to complete the injection. I decided to try for the large jaw muscle of a cheek instead of the rump. The skin is thinner and less fatty in the cheeks, so I could get the needle in faster before he launched. Wrong! He bolted as soon as I punctured the skin with the needle, but I ran along with him, pushing the plunger as we danced around the living room. More knickknacks tumbled off the one side table still standing.

"We'll know in about ten minutes if this was successful," I told the Calmers. *Whew!*

We talked of how the pig was a rescue. There are several pig rescue groups, always looking for foster or permanent homes. Usually there was no history of previous caretakers (or "non-care" takers) or of the breeding stock of origin. True potbellied pigs vary somewhat in appearance. Some look more like wild boar, with upturned snouts, bristly backs, and more or less of a potbelly. They all have swaybacks, emphasizing their pot, and are black, usually with white "boots." Others, like Charley, clearly (mostly due to size) have a lot of domestic pig in them, with splotches of unpigmented skin on the sides and back. Miniature indoor pet-type potbelly adults weigh in at thirty to sixty pounds and "large" ones tip the scale at eighty to a hundred and twenty pounds. I'd never heard of a true potbellied pig over two hundred pounds, like Charley.

Who knows what explained Charley's bull-in-a-china-shop behavior, but the current caretakers seemed to adore him. They were told by the rescue organization that the "eyeteeth" (canines or tusks) had not been pulled even though that was a usual procedure for a breeder before selling a pig. The pig had been castrated, but the vaccination history was unknown.

They were unable to get him into their car to take to a veterinary hospital, a common comment I hear from pig owners. It takes a lot of training (not so much if done at a young age) to get a pig to walk a plank from the ground into a vehicle and then have him enjoy the ride without squealing all the way down the highway.

Then there was the issue of his large size—the Calmers explained how they ended up with scratches on their arms and fell backward onto their bottoms while trying to lift his huge struggling frame into their vehicle. I chuckled with them, picturing that scene and imagining Charley then running up the porch and back inside the house or taking off down the sidewalk. The Calmers verified that Charley did all of that.

Not many hospitals will even work on potbellied pigs. I was the only "small" animal house-call veterinarian that I knew of at that time in the Sacramento region who was willing to see potbellies. Pigs are very intelligent and not easy to trick into cooperating with the stranger who would be its doctor. Veterinarians, like other sane persons, often don't want to work on an animal that makes such a racket as does a pig when restrained. The noise can be very distracting, if not downright irritating. Some say the scream is like fingernails on a blackboard. I don't mind the noise (and it helps that I have some hearing loss and can just turn off my hearing aid!), and I always prepare myself psychologically for it when calling on a pig patient. It helps to remember what my professor of porcine medicine used to remind us veterinary students: "Just think of the squealing of the pig as the sound of the cash register."

I told them that my physical examination included checking the tusks to see if they needed shearing. Charley's hooves were so over-grown that they curved outward, especially on the right front limb, where they were actually recurved. This pig definitely needed a toe-nail trim. The pig walked with a limp on that right front leg, they told me, which was the reason they called me for a home visit. That, and the fact that Charley didn't fetch the newspapers anymore.

I was concerned for injury to the spine or limb joints due to his carrying my weight around the arena. I worried that he might end up even more lame after my encounter than he was before.

Just then, Charley crashed to the floor. He was out.

I moved my medical bag over next to him, took out my stetho-scope, and listened to the chest sounds. There was such a thick wall of fat ("meat" as Mr. called it) between his skin and rib cage that I couldn't hear his heart, let alone any lung sounds. So I pushed deeply into his fleshy neck with my fingers until I could just make out the pulse of his carotid artery. Slow, but not too slow. The heav-ing of his abdominal breathing was gentle, but even.

Putting away my stethoscope, I retrieved my otoscope. A pig's ear is normally filled with the rubble of wax and debris and always appears dirty. Looking into the ear canal of a pig is like peering into an old abandoned mine shaft that is caving in. But, I looked anyway and didn't find anything unusual.

Next was to look into the eyes. Charley's cheeks and forehead were so roly-poly that the eyelids were pushed inward toward the eyeball. The eyelashes were rubbing against the cornea, causing a rivulet of tears to stain the cheek and jaw below the eye. Turning back the eyelids, I saw that the white of the eyeball (the sclera) and the normally pink inner membranes (conjunctiva) were a bright red from engorgement of the blood vessels due to irritation from the eyelashes. Peering into the innards of the eyes with the ophthalmoscope I didn't see any abnormalities except a slight blue haze of the cornea indicating irritation that could cause mild pain.

"The eyelashes are causing irritation and secondary infection of the eyes." I addressed the Calmers, "You will need to apply an eye ointment for a while to lubricate the cornea and to fight the infection."

"Is that what's making him cry all the time?" asked Mrs.

"Is that why he rubs his face on the side of the couch?" tuned Mr.

"Yes, the eyelashes rubbing inside the eye cause the tearing and irritation, even pain. But the basic cause of it is that Charley is *overweight*," giving the euphemism for obese, trying to be gentle.

Turning to his wife, Mr. said, "I told you we shouldn't be giving him pieces of our cinnamon rolls in the morning."

To which Mrs. replied, "Not just that, dear, it's the pieces of meat you barbecue with the fat and gristle still on them that you like to . . ."

"No, dearest, it's those damn cookies you use to lure him out of your garden. You know he'll do anything for a cookie. That's why he's fat."

"Well, dear," she said with her hands on her hips, swaying, with a big grin and a wink at her husband, "you will do anything for a cookie, too!"

I interjected, "Folks, folks, lots of things can make him heavy," trying to cut off at the pass what I thought might be their rising guilt. "Lots of people show love for their pet by overfeeding it. It's really very common. The important thing now is to change. If what we're doing isn't working, we need to do something else. Folks, we need to change the diet, what and how often we feed. So let's start with this—what pig feed do you give him?"

"Oh, Doctor," responded Mrs., "we buy whatever is cheapest. He goes through so much food in a month, you know."

And Mr. added, "You know, the generic food at the feed store."

"What brand? Do you have a bag of it here, so I can read the ingredients on the label?"

Mrs. answered, "No, I don't recall what brand. It's, uh, I don't know. The stuff they have in gunny sacks at the feed store."

Mr. said, "We just dump the pellets into a small garbage can we store in the garage and throw the bag away."

"Is the bag in your waste bin or somewhere where I can look at it?"

"Nope," he says, "They picked up garbage day before yesterday."

"The bags at the feed store all look alike," assured Mrs.

"Well, okay then. What is important is that you buy the best quality pig pellets you can find." I named a couple of brands and wrote them on a piece of paper for them. "Don't buy the generic feed, okay? Let me see the feed you have on hand."

Mr. led me to the garage and removed the lid of the pellet container. I reached in and grabbed a handful. Color looked okay. Then I lifted my hand to my nose. Taking a whiff, I immediately expelled air and turned away for a clearing breath.

"Whew, it smells rancid. Guys, another thing." Careful not to imply they were bad "parents," I added, "Another thing you can do to help retain the quality of the food is to store it inside the house. It gets really hot in the garage in the summer, and that can spoil the food."

"Is that why sometimes Charley turns up his nose at it when I pour some out for him?" asked Mrs.

"It's like he takes one sniff then walks away," added Mr.

"That's right. He can smell that it won't taste right. We can really help him by making sure the pellets are as fresh as can be. Keep it inside where it is cooler and keep the lid on tight."

A snort from the living room awakened me to the fact that the sedative might be wearing off and I'd best get to it.

Back at Charley's side, I palpated the skin all over his body, feeling for lumps or other abnormalities. I felt deep into his relaxed belly; all okay. I noticed that there were lines of redness and contusions on his belly, indicating he had dragged it along the ground— another effect of his being overweight. *I must remember to talk to them about portions of food.*

I took his rectal temperature. All right, 100.5° F, within normal range.

Back to his front end, I opened his mouth. Teeth okay, except for overgrown upper tusks that were cutting into his lower lips. The lower tusks were shorter, but curving outward, pressing on lower lips also. They would all need to be trimmed. I took out my wire saw (steel strands twisted tightly around each other to make ridges that cut like the teeth of a regular saw blade), wrapped it once around the circumference of one of the tusks just slightly above the gum line, put on a pair of leather gloves, and, holding each end of the wire, pulled back and forth in rhythm, sawing through the tooth. Dental dust floated up from the circuitous incision. Soon a smoky smell. I stopped, to wait a minute to let things cool down. I explained that the tooth gets hot during the procedure. Mr. reached down to feel the tooth.

"Wait, stop!" I yelled. "VERY ho—" Too late.

Mr. yelped, "Ow!" as he winced and quickly withdrew his hand. Lesson learned.

Finally, I sawed through the tusk, and it flew out of the mouth halfway across the room. Mr. fetched it, juggling it in his hands, saying, "Wow, it's still warm."

"And what are you going to do with it?" Mrs. asked.

The piece of tusk was about two inches long. I said with a smile, "Some of my clients have drilled a hole in it and strung it for a necklace or earring."

Mr. mulled something over in his head, nodding while he looked at the piece of "ivory" in the palm of his hand. He asked, "Can I have that piece of wire when you're through with it, Doc?"

After removing the other upper tusks, I cut off the protruding canine teeth of the lower jaw, having Mr. Calmer hold Charley's tongue and lower lip to one side so I wouldn't sever the soft tissue while I sawed. I took out a file and rubbed down the sharp edges of the tusks.

"Now to the hooves." I put the file away and withdrew a pair of hoof nippers, the kind you'd use on a horse. "These are sharp, so don't get your fingers in the way."

The "toenails" are very tough when overgrown, and it was going to take a while with Charley's long hooves. While I started my cutting, I told Mr. and Mrs. that the overgrowth of hooves, the painful aches in leg joints that made Charley lame, and the lack of exercise were all related in a kind of chicken-and-egg scenario with obesity. The extra weight put pressure on the joints to cause pain, and the pain and resultant lameness caused him to slow down, and the lack of exercise resulted in retention of more weight.

I began cutting away, trimming small pieces at a time, edging my way up to the quick. The end of the main blood vessel going down the inside of the hoof is accompanied by a nerve that real "quick" lets you know you've cut into it. Charley pulled his foot back with a grunt and a roll of his body when I got the hoof of the second digit just a little too short. Often I just guess where it is and try to stop short of cutting the quick.

Sometimes I can see the end of the blood vessel through a thin translucent piece of hoof I haven't yet cut through and stop there. But, inevitably, there will be at least one quick that will be hit, and it will bleed.

I got out a can of powder, a "quick-stop" as it is called. It's the same anticoagulant powder used to stop the bleeding from dehorning cattle. I sprinkled it on the bleeding end of the vessel. It usually stops bleeding immediately, and it did so this time within seconds.

I had Mr. help me flip Charley over so I could trim the other two tusks and examine the other side of his body. I had to hurry since Charley was now flinching and retracting his legs as I snipped at the last of the hooves. The sedative was wearing off.

At last, finished with the pedicure and dental work, I started brushing up the nail clippings and the cauterizing powder and asked for a cloth damp with cold water so I could wipe up the spot of blood on the carpet. They stopped me, and told me to never mind. They would clean it up. Their response was typical. People are always so nice about the mess.

I stood up and stretched. I was tired, but there was more yet to do. I still had to vaccinate and finish our discussion concerning Charley's weight problem.

I went back to my car to get the vaccines for respiratory diseases and leptospirosis. I give shots for the former since the vaccine suppresses the illness (some pigs are carriers of bacteria and break out with illness when stressed). A good reason to vaccinate for lepto is that that bacterium can be transmitted from nonhuman animals, including the pig, to people, causing serious illness. However, in my opinion, there is not much threat of leptospirosis in a house pet like a potbelly.

I loaded a hypo with yohimbe solution (a drug commonly called "Spanish fly," which is an agent sometimes used to help reverse the effects of an anesthetic or sedative) and injected it intramuscularly as soon as I could. Much better sedation-reversing drugs became available in the decade after I first saw Charley.

I told the Calmers that I would phone periodically over the next hour or two to be sure Charley woke up okay. As it turned out, it didn't take long since he was stirring and trying to gain an upright position before I left the house. While drawing up the vaccines into syringes and injecting them, I engaged the Calmers in discussion regarding diet.

"You know, potbellied pigs are house pets, not pigs you fatten up for market. When you feed leftovers . . ."

"Oh no," interrupted Mrs., "it's not just 'leftovers.' We cook especially for Charley. If we're barbecuing a steak and a potato, we throw one on for him, too."

"We baked him a cake for his birthday," added Mr.

Spinning that idea over in my mind, I pictured Charley's snout covered with frosting and candles sticking out his nostrils and between his lips. "Yes, I know you love Charley, and only want the best for him. However . . . However, to keep him healthy we need to do what is best for him. Love can kill. Especially overfeeding him."

"He likes the food we give him," Mr. chimed in.

"He'll eat whatever we give him and be quite happy," Mrs. informs.

"But that's the problem. He's an omnivore, like we are. He'll eat all you give him, at least until he's full. In the wilds his ancestors foraged for food by rooting up whatever roots and vegetables and grubs they could get. And they ran around the Vietnamese jungles getting their exercise. Charley is bred differently. He actually needs a lot less food than you probably would guess. How many cups of pig chow pellets do you feed daily?"

Mr. replied, "Some days we don't give him any, just our 'leftover' spaghetti or corncobs, or whatever."

"And cabbage, or cooked carrots, celery, peas." Mrs. added assurance and with an apologetic tone, "Good vegetables!"

Feeling a little frustrated, but also amused, I said, "I'm sure it's all good stuff and not spoiled. But my point is that all the protein, vitamins, and minerals that Charley needs are in good quality pellets. He doesn't need any other food. If he is fed exclusively pellets, nothing else, he'll do just fine. All the other extra food makes him unhealthy."

"I guess you're right. He is too fat. We don't want him to have runny eyes and rub his belly raw on the ground."

"And we don't want him to get achy joints like you said. My doctor told me that if I lost weight I would have fewer aches and pains in my knees and feet."

I jumped on that. "Yes, just like you, and me by the way," tapping my tummy. "He would be better off by losing a few pounds. We want to get him to where his eyelids don't scratch his eyes and make them water anymore. But, just like what we would do for ourselves, we need to wean him off of food gradually. He will beg for food at first, but we have to be strict about what we feed him."

With a sad look, Mrs. says, "Be cruel to be kind."

"Love him enough . . ." Mr. trailed off. "What shall we feed him and how often?"

I nodded, "Normal sized potbellied pigs can get by with only one-half to one cup of pellets per day. Since Charley is not a normal-sized potbelly, he maybe should get about two or two and a half cups per day. But it sounds like Charley is used to several times that volume, I should imagine. So we'll start out by giving him four cups, two in the morning and two at night."

"Okay. How many pancakes can we give him when we cook 'em on Sundays?"

"He loves them with molasses syrup, and strawberries when they're in season."

Gag. A little overboard! Choking, but laughing at the same time, I said, "Okay, folks. No pancakes. And, and, no syrup. None. Nada. No cakes, no spaghetti, just pellets."

"But that will be so boring."

"Yeah, I wouldn't want to eat just pellets."

In my mind I agreed with them, but I continued, "You are not a pig, and Charley is not a pig you are fattening up for market."

In unison, but with downcast expressions, "Oh."

I continued, "When he gets grumpy from lack of food and terrorizes the living room, ignore him. But you can treat him when he quiets down and does what you want. Reward him with a slice or two of apple, a carrot, or three or four grapes when he behaves. That way he won't feel totally deprived. And you'll be training him. Pigs are very intelligent."

Almost in unison, "He sure is. He knows we're suckers for handouts. He pushes against our table legs until he gets some of our biscuits and gravy. Okay, what else?"

"Patience is primary. You have to reduce the volume of food, pellets, slowly. Once a month, cut back on the amount you feed him, but only by a little bit. For example, if this month you feed two cups in a.m. and two cups in p.m., feed two cups in morning and one and four-fifths in the evening next month. Cut down slowly, and let's give him eighteen months to get his weight down. And, another thing. If you do give him a 'treat' or he gets into something he shouldn't, cut back on the amount of pellets you give that evening. Food is food."

"I will try my best, Doc," Mrs. stated, "but I'll have to watch my husband too." Blushing, she added, "No, not what he eats, but what he feeds Charley."

Chuckling, Mr. said, "Well, maybe that would be good for me, too. And I could chase him around the yard to give him some exercise."

"And chase him out of my garden!" added Mrs.

We all had a good laugh imagining that. We discussed some of the details a little more, and how long to treat the eyes with antibiotic ointment. "Reward with a couple of grapes or celery stalk when he lets you do it. Phone and let me know Charley's progress. Call me out for a visit in eighteen to twenty-four months to trim hooves again if needed." A plan was born.

A year had passed when I received a phone call from the Mrs.

"Hello, Doctor. Charley's eyes have stopped running and his belly doesn't drag on the ground. He seems a lot more energetic, too."

Another voice on the line, "And who'd a thought he would have more energy with less food?"

"That's great! I'm really pleased to hear of your progress. I guess he's lost enough weight that his leg joints don't ache as much, so he feels more like moving around. Let's make that appointment for the nail trim check and physical exam for six months from now. And you just continue what you are doing. I'm so glad to hear Charley's better."

"And," says Mrs., "my husband didn't lose any of his belly, but he has toned up chasing Charley."

"And Charley sure can run fast," adds Mr. with a belly laugh. "We call out 'Whoopee,' remembering how you rode on his back that day you were here. He just squeals with delight running around the living room knocking things over faster than he ever did before!"

15

Three Little Pigs

None went to market.

Petunia

A cute little piggy that went for walks around the grounds and rose garden of the Capitol building.

Her "dad" lived in an upstairs apartment a few blocks from the seat of the California Legislature. Every morning "Dad" Tim trussed 'Tunia up in a harness and hooked it with a dog leash. That is, every morning except on days he was booming forth his melodious baritone voice onstage at the San Francisco Opera House.

But, funny thing, Tim didn't look like the prototypical opera singer. No barrel chest, no beard, nor was he of short or average stature. No, he stretched to at least six foot three inches tall and was rail thin. Whenever I saw him he wore a tight T-shirt and khaki shorts exposing his protruding ribs and matchstick legs.

Petunia, on the other hand, barely reached two feet tall, not even reaching Tim's mid-shins. The two of them, tall pole-like Tim and his tiny squat Petunia, made quite an unusual appearing pair as he walked her like a dog along the sidewalks of downtown Sacramento. Tim even carried plastic bags with which to scoop Petunia's poop.

I met Petunia and Tim on a gorgeous Tahoe-blue-sky day in spring. I squeezed my car into a small paved lot next door to the apartment building. The sign read RESIDENT PARKING ONLY. I hoped Tim had a placard I could place on my dashboard so my car wouldn't be towed away.

The lower level of the building was a small mom-and-pop market. There was a door leading up to the apartments to the left of the store, but the entrance to Tim's pad was on the parking side of the building. The stairs to his apartment were wooden steps with a steel railing that led up to a small landing at his doorstep. As I climbed the stairway lugging my medical bag, I wondered if he had to carry his pig up and down the stairs on his comings and goings. That question was answered momentarily.

I heard someone from down below call my name as I ascended the stairs.

"Dr. MacVean, I assume." There was Tim with Petunia in tow coming along the sidewalk. He waved and said, "Wait at the top. The door is locked." He gave a little whistle as he reached the bottom of the stairs, and Petunia immediately started bounding her way up the steps with ease. *Clearly, no need to carry that little girl.*

Later, when I started in on a mini lecture regarding how stairs, especially going down, could be rough on his pig's shoulder and knee and ankle joints, Tim assured me he knew of that potential and always carried her down the steps. He also mentioned that they were moving to another apartment that was on the ground floor. He added, "The new apartment has a small backyard, so 'Tunia can root outside sometimes instead of tossing our rugs all over the place."

Tim unlocked the wooden door that was painted a subdued violet color. He ushered me in as Petunia sniffed at my pant legs, smearing a little snot as she read of the dogs and cats I'd seen earlier in the day. Apparently chuffed, she lifted her tiny snout with one last sniff and then tiptoed her way toward a curtained room off to the side of the living room.

The apartment was artfully decorated. Colorful throw rugs on dark walnut flooring, quilts over the dark leather coach and easy chair, reproductions of Miró and Picasso paintings hung on a wall, a multi-hued stained glass lampshade covered the lights over a blond-knotty-pine dinner table. An aroma of lemon filled the air, as if the table had been rubbed with a citrus oil. Rich-textured curtains hung at exits to a hallway and the kitchen off the main room. Overhead lighting was recessed, with spotlights aimed at the paintings. There was a high-end record player and stereo speakers on a cream-colored cabinet against one wall. The room was well lit by windows at the back of the main room. It all was strikingly memorable to me. It was a living space of comfort, and I asked about it.

"Ah, yes. The decorative touches are my partner John's tasteful doings. The music is mine." Then he proceeded to tell me he was a lead baritone for the San Francisco Opera. John, he said, was a chef at one of the restaurants nearby. They also had an apartment in the Castro district of San Francisco. Tim would stay there when he had continual work at the Opera, and John would take care of Petunia while he was gone.

Dishes rattled off behind the curtain to the kitchen. I set my bag down on a chair next to the table and pointed toward the noise of pottery clinking. "I guess that's John getting a meal together."

"No, it's 'Tunia rooting among her water and food bowls, looking for a drink and snack. But they're empty since you told me not to feed or water her this morning. I'll go get her." And off he went parting the drapes hanging at the archway to the kitchen.

I pulled out the smallest of my hoof nippers, blood-stop powder, syringe with needle, and the bottles of sedative and reversing agent and arranged them on the floor in a well-lit area near the windows.

Petunia ambled out of the kitchen, reluctantly moving ahead of Tim's herding motions. She let out a little squeal. I supposed she was disappointed at no morsel in her dish. Her harness had been removed. She made a beeline for my bag and stood up on her hind legs with front legs on the chair edge. She sniffed my bag and shoved it with her snout.

"Ha, Tim, I think she discovered with that good smeller of hers that I have pet treats in my bag." I got down on my knees and put my arms around her. As I did so, I noticed a sweet smell and a hint of lavender. "She sure smells good. I like the touch of lavender."

"We bathed her yesterday." And with a smile he added, "Just for you!"

"Really. Many pigs hate bathing."

"'Tunia actually looks forward to it. We just walk her into the shower and lather her up with baby shampoo to which we've added a couple drops of lavender oil."

"That's a new one on me."

Still on the floor on my knees, I lifted Petunia to get some idea of her weight. *Uh, uh, heavy little thing! Around forty-five to fifty pounds.* Little potbellies may be short, but they are compact and usually weigh more than a dog of comparable height. I lifted a lip and saw that her tusks were no longer than the rest of her teeth. *No need for a tusk trim.* I didn't really expect that she would since she was only about two years of age, at least a full year from full mature growth. Also, females are much less likely to require tusk trimming than males.

I leaned back a little, hugging her to my chest, and rubbed her belly. She didn't seem to mind the restraint and appeared to like the tummy touch. Also, I took a good look at her hooves. "Well, Tim, there is not a lot to take off her toenails. Probably because they're worn by the daily walks on concrete." Then I took hold of one of her front legs. She immediately squealed and struggled to get out of my hold. I let her go. She ran a few steps away from me and turned her head with her eyelids and forehead wrinkled up into a scowl.

"She does not like her feet touched. I can do most anything to her, but her feet are definitely off limits."

With a sigh, I replied, "I know. That's often the case with pigs unless they're trained to accept it at an early age. I'll give her a light sedative injection so we can get the trimming done."

"That won't be necessary, Doc. I can make sure she's quite docile for your procedure."

"And how might that be?"

He ambled over to the stereo turntable, lifted the tone arm and gently placed the stylus onto the black vinyl of a record. Melodic symphonic music began to flood the room.

He winked at me and took in a deep breath. His thin chest expanded like the ribs of an accordion. What came out of his mouth were rich lofty tones of a lush aria from a Verdi composition. The vocal music enriched the air. I was stunned at his modulating control from stirring softness to expansive explosion of sound settling into the quiet of a lake smooth as a mirror. Calm, soothing.

Then I heard a thud. Petunia had plopped over on her side halfway onto her back with legs straight out in front of her. Her eyelids fluttered and closed. She was out like a light.

She was in a hypnotic state. *Tim's singing! She responds with slumber as if she were a baby listening to a good-night lullaby.*

No problemo. Trimming her hooves was a piece of cake. I came close to the quick of one of her nails, and she didn't even flinch. It was easy giving her the once-over examination and the vaccine shots.

As soon as I was through with the vet work, I stood up. "I'm done. That was the easiest pedicure I've ever given to a pig."

Tim ended the aria on a long bass note. Within not even a minute of the end of his singing, Petunia stirred. Her curly eyelashes fluttered. She rolled over and stood up. She shook her body a couple of times like a wet dog after a shower. Getting her bearings, as if nothing unusual had happened, she deftly tiptoed over to sniff my bag again.

Oh, what harm in it. I unzipped my bag, took out one of the vitamin dog treats and handed it to her. She crumbled it in her mouth and leisurely gulped a couple of times and then pointed her snout at my bag as if she were Charles Dickens's Oliver saying "More, sir."

Tim and I chuckled. He said he would have her favorite treat, Cheerios, available for my next visit.

When I got down to the bottom of the steps and saw my car I realized I'd forgotten to get the temporary parking permit placard from Tim. I was pleased to see my car had not been towed away. I looked at the car's front window. No paper ticket under the windshield wiper. *Whew, I got away with it again. Who polices these parking spots anyway?* I felt cheerful, looking forward to later visits and hearing more opera and a snoring pig.

Caesar

This fine potbellied pig was the monarch of the turf at Richard Land's house.

I was at the home to perform a physical examination and to update vaccinations for the Land family's pet, who lived a cushy life in their regime. And they were the first to admit to that. Subservient they were.

"Hi, I'm Dick and this is my wife, Betty. Come on in 'n meet our boy, Caesar." They led me through the living room, through a dining room, through the kitchen, and into a sunroom at the back of the house. This was Caesar's room.

All along the back wall was a bank of windows, but too high for Caesar to see more than the overhang of the roof, sky, and the top limbs of a couple of trees. The wall was south facing, so plenty of daylight streamed into his room, especially in winter. In one corner of the wall stood a large electric fan. No doubt there were plenty of cooling breezes in summer since, in addition to the standing fan, there was an overhead ceiling fan. To the left were two plastic bins containing dog toys, both rubber squeaky kinds and stuffed animals. Near the wall to the right was a double-size dog bed with a rumpled heap of blankets over one side of the bed, trailing off onto the linoleum floor.

I commented, "Looks like Caesar sleeps in cozy comfort, with all those blankets and the soft mattress." While raising my eyebrows in wonderment, I added, "Where did you find such an oversized dog bed?"

Betty answered with a prideful smile, "We had a small dog bed when we first got him twelve years ago. But he grew so big; we had to get something larger. So I bought two of the largest dog beds I could find and sewed them together with leather strips. But he outgrew that. What you see now is four large dog beds knitted into one."

Why not just buy a large mattress? "But there are no ridges in the middle. How did you . . ."

Betty continued, "I simply slit the edges that were to come together, removed some of the stuffing, and stitched it back."

"Caesar sleeps like a baby."

A rather large baby. "Okay, nice job. Where is your baby?"

"Probably out back." Dick pointed to the door in the left wall—a door that had the bottom half of it hinged to swing out like a heavy-duty double-wide doggy door. It was padded at the bottom, like weather stripping.

Dick led me out into what was called a backyard. The grass was sparse and uneven, no doubt from indentations from Caesar's hooves and from his rooting for worms or grubs. No Caesar.

As we walked back inside Dick said, "He's probably watching TV."

TV?

We marched through a hallway with well-worn flooring to a bedroom halfway down the corridor. Off on one side of the room was a low-slung overstuffed couch with an overstuffed pig stretched out on it. Caesar looked to be at least a couple hundred pounds. His color was white pink with small brown spots. He was quite attentively looking at the television on the opposite side of the small room. There was a love seat next to the couch.

Dick explained. "He's really smart. I think he knows what is happening on the programs he likes to watch. We set it to Animal Planet or, if he grunts loudly like he wants us to change channels, we tune to Discovery or National Geographic." Other times he wanted the music channels. He would stare off into space as if in reverie whenever classical music was played. He didn't care much for rock. Motioning toward the love seat, Dick added, "We often join him for 'family time.' We used to sit with him, but he's gotten too big for us to join him on the couch."

"Such a life!" I said. "I can do some of the physical examination with him lying on the couch, but I'll need him to stand up and walk for the rest of the exam."

I walked over to Caesar and held my hand out in front of his snout so he could get a good whiff of me. He barely sniffed. I spoke to him about needing his cooperation for the exam. He raised his snout in a way I interpreted as snooty and an "I can't be bothered" attitude, as if to say "Do what you must, but don't interrupt my program."

I got out my stethoscope and otoscope/ophthalmoscope and proceeded with the exam. I didn't bother to get out the rectal thermometer. I was sure he would object to that distraction. Anyway, he checked out fine in all respects. A little tearing at the corner of the eyes, but no more than usual for an overweight "potbellied" pig. While conducting the exam, I inquired about feeding. The Lands' answers were nowhere near as ebullient as the menu for chubby

Charley. I gave a shortened feeding regime lecture to Dick and Betty since they were pretty much up to speed in that area.

I took out one of the vitamin treats to lure Caesar up for the rest of the exam. He wouldn't budge. I tried nudging him. No go.

"Well, I'll try to palpate his internal organs from the sides of his belly." He didn't cooperate well, nudging my hands away from his side by pushing with his snout. *At least you're paying attention to me.*

Dick offered a solution. "He loves grapes. I'll get some from the freezer. Bet he gets up then."

Betty went off to the kitchen and returned holding a small aluminum bucket that contained a few frozen grapes. When she swung the container back and forth, the grapes made a rattling sound. It worked. Caesar slowly rolled over the edge of the sofa and stood. He grunted, but didn't move any closer to the bucket.

"We need to bring the treats to him. He doesn't come to us. He actually prefers that we hand-feed him." She looked at me and moved her head back and forth. "I know, I know. He has us well trained."

"All right, then, you hand him one grape at a time, and I'll finish my exam while he stands here."

Betty held out a grape in the palm of her hand right up to Caesar's lips. He curled his lip and sucked the grape into his mouth and chewed it up. Betty proceeded this way with the next dozen grapes while I pushed up on Caesar's pendulous belly to palpate for any abnormalities. Everything was fine until I moved to his rear. There was a stringy object of some sort dangling from his anus. I grabbed hold of it and pulled.

Caesar bolted. I was left holding a wad of grass-like material stuck together with smelly stool. The Lands guffawed. Caesar stood at the doorway looking back at me with the unmistakable look of indignation and a snort that I heard as "How dare you?"

Caesar then ambled off down the hall. Dick shouted, "Hurry

up. Come on. You've got to see this," and went off along the hallway after his pig, leaving me holding my stringy mess.

Finding no convenient place to dump the load, I followed down the hall holding the green and brown clump in one hand, using the other hand to keep it from dripping onto the floor. I reached the room at the other end of the hall just in time to see Caesar walk up a wide wooden ramp from the floor to a wooden platform that had a hole cut out toward the back of it. Caesar reached the top, turned completely around, and faced me while he squatted and dumped a load down the hole. Standing full up, he wiggled his rear end a little, shaking off a last clump. Then he turned back around to the toilet tank and flushed the handle with his snout!

As calm as could be, he turned around and moved down the ramp with hips rolling as if he were a fashion model in a slow stately stride across a catwalk. With head aloof, he brushed by me as if I was not there and headed back down the hall toward the TV room.

While feeling a little humiliated holding the smelly prize in my hands, I also felt impressed with Caesar's performance. I heard Dick say, "What did you think of that, huh? I built the ramp and trained him when he was young. Of course I've had to keep enlarging and reinforcing the ramp and platform as he got larger."

I must have stimulated his need to go to the bathroom by tugging on that wad of stuff that dangled from his bum. Just like dogs, pigs will sometimes eat a clump of grass that will end up passing all the way through.

Dick was grinning. "You can put that stuff down in the waste-basket over there near the sink."

The basket was lined with a plastic grocery store bag. *Easy disposal.* I chatted with Dick while I squeezed soap out of a dispenser and washed my hands. "You did a good job with the toilet training. Pigs learn quickly. That is really clever. How did you get the idea? What was your training method?"

"I read in a pig magazine about some guy who built the same kind of toilet 'bowl' for his pig. I thought, 'Wow, what a great idea. I'm gonna do it.' I've done a little cabinetry on my job, so building it was not difficult. Training was easy once we discovered what reward worked best for him."

"Rewarding is the best. When he does what you want, you give him his reward treat. What was it?"

"Oreo cookies! He would do anything for an Oreo. But we started using grapes, a healthier treat, once he got larger."

"Good. He's got the potty routine down well. He doesn't even have to go outside to relieve himself."

"Of course we have our own toilet in the master bedroom. He stays out of there," Dick said with a chuckle. "There are a few other tricks we trained him to do, but now he's too old. Set in his ways."

I responded, "Maybe he is still capable of learning new ways, if he thinks it's in his best interests. Caesar seems like the type that will choose on his own what he wants to learn, now that you have established that he is king of his domain. He doesn't need to please you anymore. He pleases himself."

Dick nodded with enthusiasm. "Man, you can say that again! He's figured out how to push our buttons."

"He might just be ignoring you when you try new things now. Of course grapes are not quite the incentive as Oreos for sure. I'm not convinced that 'you can't teach an old dog new tricks' applies to pigs. They're smarter than that. I know one guy that taught his old porcine companion to walk a labyrinth."

"You have a point there. He is the emperor." Dick had me walk around with him so he could show me the front of the bathroom door. There hung a handwritten sign that read CAESAR's THRONE.

Betty was still standing in the hallway. She added, "When he was young he potty trained immediately. We taught him to sit, stay, fetch, and shake hands. A smart little pig."

I smiled and said, "Ha, I know some relatives of mine that aren't that smart!" We all laughed, nodding heads in agreement.

I asked them to lead me to a table with good lighting, so I could fill out the paperwork. We all went off to the kitchen, and I sat down at the dinette.

"Caesar's gait is excellent. No lameness, no swollen joints; and his hooves don't need trimming."

Dick then informed me, "Caesar does a good job of rubbing his hooves down himself. He digs in our backyard like a dog burying a bone."

"Ha, so that's why. Okay. His tusks don't protrude beyond his lips, so no need to cut the tusks. Also, I really don't want to expose him to the risk of using an injectable sedative at his age. I don't see the need to boost his vaccines. You had said earlier on the phone that he doesn't see other pigs or dogs. His breathing seems fine, and there is no snot on his nose like he might have if he had a respiratory problem. Unless he shows signs of illness, I don't think I need to see him again for another couple of years."

When we concluded our business Betty remarked, "Thank you, Dr. MacVean, for your kind assessment." With a chuckle she added, "And I'm sorry you ended up with a handful of poop."

We all laughed.

A memorable visit to a crown monarch in his pigdom.

Punchy

"He's a scrapper," said Mrs. Susan Salton.

I was warned.

"Don't think it will be a problem," I said as I eyed the small potbelly standing in the middle of the backyard." He was a white and black five-year-old neutered male that stood only slightly over two feet tall and looked no more than sixty to seventy pounds in weight. "With your husband's help it should be fine."

"Oh, you don't know Punchy. Got his name from using me and James as punching bags as a young'un. He was ornery to start"

Her husband, James, nodded in agreement. He was a stocky, muscular five feet eight. He wasn't much for words. Susan did most of the talking.

Addressing me, Susan said, "I got Cousin Henry to agree to come help hold. He'll be here shortly." Addressing her husband, she advised, "James, do whatever the vet wants." Addressing me again, she said, "We have a six-foot-high wooden fence, strong, all around our backyard, so Punchy ain't goin' nowhere."

"We probably won't need the extra muscle for that li'l piggy. James, do you have a couple of five-gallon buckets we can use?"

"I have one, not two. But I also have a galvanized steel wash-basin."

"Ah, even better, in case we need to herd him around to where we want him. For now, let's go get hold of him." I knew we would need to wrestle Punchy to the ground so I could hog-tie him. Susan insisted that no injectable sedative be used since a previous doctor at a vet hospital had "'killed" her other potbellied pig, Judy, with such a shot. I thought of telling her how rare that is, but my canceling thought was that it would be easy to handle that little pig.

I had my rope handy as James and I approached.

Punchy was super alert, floppy ears now erect. He lowered his head and snorted, with nostrils flaring like those of a raging bull. He looked like he was going to charge us.

"Okay, James, get behind him, and I'll take the front. Move slowly. When I give the signal, grab his hind legs and I'll grab the front end."

I heard Susan sputter, "Like a rat's ass you will."

James and I moved together to squeeze the distance between us and Punchy. Just as I gave the signal to pounce, Punchy bolted right for me, knocking me tumbling. Pain sparked through my back and rear when I hit the ground. Their backyard was mostly dirt, hard-packed beneath, but loose dust on the surface.

"I got hold of one leg when he rammed into you, but he slipped loose. He ran around to the side of the house."

I stood, picked up my rope, and brushed off the dust. "Maybe that's a good thing." *Much narrower space than the backyard.* "Let's get the buckets. You slip around behind him with the basin and I'll use the pail over his snout to back him up to you. Then when he is trapped, we'll grab him."

I caught Susan out of the corner of my eye slowly shaking her head back and forth. *So little faith.*

James did manage to slide by Punchy and get behind him. Punchy had a wary eye on him all the way.

Holding up the basin, James yelled, "Okay, I'm ready."

I lowered the pail to snout level and approached. I kept legs planted firmly with each step, so I had better traction to keep from falling backward if "attacked" again. With a bucket over his snout and covering his eyes a pig will usually back up. Then we would have him in our bucket "vise."

I got the pail over his head, and Punchy backed up. But that was just a ruse. That clever little guy was just getting traction of his own, and he proved to be stronger than I thought. As soon as his rear end touched the metal basin and before I could shout "Grab him!" Punchy moved his head sideways enough to dislodge the bucket from around his head and plowed his little legs so fast they were a blur as he rushed past me. James and my arms were flailing. Empty handed. Punchy opened his mouth squealing at the top of his lungs as he ran out of sight to the other side of the house where the doghouse was that he often slept in.

Punchy squealed and Susan laughed, while James and I inhaled dust and coughed.

A man about the same height as James, and just as burly, opened the wooden gate behind James and entered the yard. Cousin Henry had arrived.

I don't like having to play cowboy rounding up a patient, but at least I had help. *Reinforcements for the tug-of-war about to begin.*

I tied a slipknot on the end of my rope and made a noose. My idea was to slip the loop over Punchy's snout when he opened his mouth to squeal at us. Piggy would back up and the noose would tighten around his upper jaw and I'd have him tugging one way and me the other way. James and Henry could then grab Punchy, turn him onto his side, and I could hog-tie a front leg to his hind legs.

Anyway, that was my plan.

With a smirk on her face, Susan chuckled, "You gonna lasso him? Good luck!"

I would need it. *Now, if Punchy would only open his mouth wide enough. . .*

We moved the doghouse to help block exit from the small rectangular area on that side of the house. The three of us surely could act as a barrier for the rest of the space. We all lined up so Punchy was cornered. But quicker than a bullet train, that little pig railed at us and bolted at the plastic doghouse and brushed it aside in the blink of an eye. Off he ran, back to the other side of the house where we first thought we'd cornered him.

Susan slapped her hand on her thigh and laughed, and laughed, and laughed. Boy, did I feel sheepish. My face turned red.

Once things settled down and we started to think about our next strategy for capturing that tornado called a pig, Susan offered some iced tea.

"Naw, I want to finish the job. Other appointments are on my list today." The challenge Punchy presented was as much mental as physical. I attempted to convince Susan of the value of a sedative, but she would have none of it. Of course I would still need to restrain the pig long enough to give the injection. *So what is the point?*

THREE LITTLE PIGS

To make it easier to trim the hooves and tusks, I reassured myself. I wished I had a squeeze chute to herd Punchy into. Then the light-bulb went off in my head.

"Hey, James, do you have a large piece of plywood or siding or gate or something we could use as a barrier? That way we could all together hold it up and squeeze Punchy up against the fence."

"Nope. Can't think of anything we could use for that."

"Okay, well, I'll just have to be faster at getting the noose on him." *As a last resort.*

The three of us lined up side by side. We crouched in a position to better make a stab at grabbing Punchy as he tried to get by us, just in case I was unsuccessful with the lasso. Punchy faced us, his rear up against the fence gate.

I approached, and Punchy opened his mouth in a squeal that sounded like a kid screaming at the top of his lungs. I slipped the noose over his snout and tightened the rope. Sure enough, he tried to back up. I stepped back and tugged.

"Grab him now," I shouted.

James and Henry quickly pounced on the pig while me and Punchy played out our tug-of-war.

As soon as the men had Punchy on his side, I ran up and quickly wrapped my end of the rope over his body and around the hind leg on the down side and then looped it around a front leg and back to the other rear leg and tied them all together. I felt as proud of myself as if I'd won a prize at a rodeo calf-tying competition.

With Punchy struggling to get loose and the men grappling to hold him down, we kicked up a cumulonimbus cloud of dust. Punchy bawled his high-pitched wail at the top of his lungs the whole time I tried nipping the hooves. James and Henry tried to hold his squirming legs.

Then, bursting through the gate and into the dust were a group of three uniformed men. Cops. One of them yelled, "Stop! Onto the ground." And another grabbed Henry's arm away from the body he was struggling to hold down.

"What the . . ." I yelled.

The dust was settling.

The policemen stopped short. They saw we had a pig in our grasp. They started laughing, realizing the mistake.

"What's going on?" I said. Punchy was tied, so I rose to find out why we were being accosted by cops. The squealing had quieted, but was still fairly loud.

The head guy explained that a neighbor called 911 to report a kid was screaming his head off. Being physically abused. "The lady even described the gate we could use to get into the yard to intervene."

It is for sure that a pig squealing could sound like a kid being beaten. Susan came up just then and joined in the explanation to the policemen. Of course, she wanted to know which "nosy" neighbor reported it. The cops wouldn't satisfy her curiosity, but did let us know they were satisfied nothing unlawful or immoral was going on. They filled out a report sheet and left.

With James and Henry holding the legs as best as they could, I finished the hoof trims. The tusks were short and didn't need to be sawed off at this time. By the time the last clipping was made, we were all dripping with sweat.

I untied Punchy and stood up. He wandered off slowly toward the back, grunting, but glancing back at us as if to be sure we were not following. The loud noise had finally stopped assaulting our ears. That squeal sure can sound and feel as annoying as chalk scratching on a blackboard. I turned to Susan and said, "I could use that glass of iced tea right now."

We all sat with a glass of cold tea in hand at a picnic table in the yard and sipped—chugalugged in my case. We talked of the gendarme invasion and the screaming "kid." Susan mostly laughed.

James and Henry mostly commented on the scratches they'd received from Punchy's flailing hooves while trying to restrain the pig.

I was pretty quiet. I didn't mention how I wasn't fond of how I had to traumatize the poor pig to do my job. Visually Punchy needed a hoof trim. But, considering how fast and sure he could run around escaping our attempts to grab him, he didn't need the trim functionally. I did resolve, then and there, to not take on any more patients wherein I would have to resort to hog-tying.

The iced tea was good. But I did ask Susan to put a slice of lemon in it for me. To cover up the bitter taste in my mouth, and to help wash down the dust.

Pigs as patients have been fulfilling in many ways, in spite of the sometimes difficult situations I've gone through with them. They are intelligent and interesting companions. They're loved dearly by the special people who take care of them. The squealing has not been merely "the sound of the cash register" as my porcine medicine professor had suggested. No, for me, it has been the bleating expression of experiences. High-quality, unforgettable experiences.

III
Transitions

"An animal's eyes have the power to speak a great language."
—Martin Buber, *I and Thou*

"If having a soul means being able to feel love and loyalty and gratitude, then animals are better off than a lot of humans."
—James Herriot, *All Creatures Great and Small*

"We are all visitors to this time, this place. We are just passing through. Our purpose here is to observe, to learn, to grow, to love . . . and then we return home."
—Australian Aboriginal proverb

16

The Wailing

'Twas the night the animals spoke.

My wife, Marsha, was along for the ride and to assist me with my patient if needed. We had eaten dinner, and the rain had stopped; so we thought it might be a pleasant ride into the countryside. But I had an ulterior motive for asking her along. She is good with people, and I hoped she could help calm down the woman who phoned me. Mrs. Sheridan was hysterical when she called me to come out and put Diamond to sleep. She said her nine-year-old malamute refused to eat or drink, could not get up, and was in a lot of pain.

It had rained all day, so the curvy dirt road into the Double D Ranch was treacherous that night. The road looked like it had never been graded, as the grooves for the wheels were more like arroyos than ruts. There were pockets of muddy water that loomed like lakes. My pickup, even in four-wheel drive, slid from side to side as it forged on through. On one turn the vehicle slipped out of the grooves and skidded toward a twisted oak that stood guard at that curve. The bark showed scar slashes from prior encounters with solid objects that had left the road. Fortunately, I missed the tree and slid back into the furrows. It was a long "driveway" and had to be taken slowly. With having to stop for gas on the way and then the rebellious road, I was late for the house call.

"Where have you been?" Mrs. S. shouted. "I thought you would *never* get here. What were you doing? My dog is dying. He's in pain!" Her frenzied tone became even more frenetic in response to my explanations of why I was delayed. "You don't care about my Diamond. You just take your own damned time."

Her husband stood there, seeming lost and staring down at the floor. Marsha stepped forward, interrupting Mrs. S.'s tirade. She led the Mrs. into the kitchen, talking about needing a cup of tea. It worked like magic, diverting the frantic woman.

Mr. Sheridan then spoke up and apologized for his wife's misplaced anger. "We've been under a lot of stress lately, with me out of a job and not being able to meet all the bills." He added, as if I might be worried, "Oh, it's okay. I have the cash for your fee. I want you to do what is best for Diamond."

"You know, it's quite all right. I often see people angry about losing a pet. I don't take it personally. And I sure can understand the grief and other pressures contributing to the anger."

I did not add that there was some anger on my part, too. They did not take care of Diamond's leg a year ago when I last saw him— when Mr. S. did have a job. At that time the swelling that was causing some mild lameness was confined to a bone (radius) in the lower part of the left front leg, near the elbow. I had stuck a needle into the swelling and pulled a small portion of tissue up into a syringe. The pathologist I sent the sample to identified the lesion as an aggressive bone cancer called osteosarcoma, a scourge much more common in large-boned dogs than other breeds. What upset me was that if they had taken my advice and had the leg amputated at that time, the cancer would have been eliminated and not have a chance to spread. Diamond would get along just fine on three legs.

We were standing on a wet spongy throw rug near the front door at the entrance to the living room. It was apparent that water had run down the slope from the barn to their front doorstep and into the room. The air smelled of barn effluent. The living room floorboards appeared dry in the area where Diamond lay. There was a squeegee-like apparatus with a long handle leaning up against a wall.

Mr. S. noticed my looking at the surroundings, "The rain was really heavy. Poured cats and dogs. Flooded the living room. Diamond plunked himself down onto the middle of the floor. He wouldn't, well, couldn't move. So we cleaned up around him. He's pretty much where he first fell down. We haven't been able to move him without his crying out in pain."

It was sad to see this superb animal lying there, his breath a shallow panting. It was cold. "Please close the door. And can you get another lamp in here? It's too dark for me to see and evaluate Diamond."

"Sorry, Doc. We're leaving the door open to dry out. We don't have another lamp, but I'll get a flashlight." Mr. S. then went off to the kitchen.

Diamond looked part wild canine with wolf-gray-colored haircoat and long big-boned legs. The mask markings on his head and muzzle gave him a mysterious look. He weighed over eighty pounds and looked even larger with his heavy fur and thick undercoat.

I knelt beside Diamond. His eyes told me he was ready to go. There is a certain look in animal's eyes when it is their time, as if saying "Please ease my pain. Release me." His whole leg was swollen with edema, and an ulcer had developed in the skin over the elbow. I tried as tenderly as possible to examine the leg. The radius and likely the bone next to it (the ulna) were fractured, a common outcome due to the fragile nature of bone that has been eaten away by cancer. The dog showed signs of emphysema, difficulty expelling air from his lungs between panting spells. It was due, no doubt in my mind, to spread of the cancer from bone through his bloodstream to his air passages. Poor Diamond was in pain, couldn't walk, and could barely breathe. He had to be euthanized.

When Mr. S. returned with the flashlight, I stood up and informed him, "It is time to let him go. Don't let him suffer anymore."

"I thought so. And so does my wife. I'll stay here and help you, but Sally does not want to be present." He started toward the kitchen. "I'll tell her."

I took out my euthanasia kit and filled a syringe with the lethal formula. I would not need a sedative for Diamond. He was a sweet dog the last time I visited here, and I was sure he would not be inclined to move. I'd simply find a vein in one of his rear legs for the injection.

All three came out of the kitchen. I had Mr. sign the euthanasia authorization form while Mrs. knelt down and petted Diamond good-bye. When Mrs. stood up, she was crying, and wiping her eyes with her apron. She looked at me and said, "Thank you." She turned and walked back into the kitchen. Marsha said she would wait in the truck, then patted Diamond and walked out the front door. Mr. S. said he wanted to stay and hold his dog.

I knelt on the floor next to Diamond and applied the tourniquet above a vein near the hock (ankle) of a rear leg. Mr. shone the flashlight on the area I pointed to. I couldn't really see the bulge of the vein through the thick fur, but I could feel it with my fingers. I guided the needle in and then pulled back on the plunger of the syringe to see blood come up into the syringe, verifying that the needle was in the vein. I loosened the tourniquet and slowly pushed the plunger, feeding the solution into Diamond's body. By the time half the liquid was in, Diamond's breathing stopped. When three quarters of it had been given, the fur on his chest that had swayed in rhythm with his heartbeat stopped moving.

Then, as the plunger reached the bottom of the syringe, a strange, mysterious, miraculous thing happened. The Sheridans' other two dogs, which were out near the barn, began to howl. At the same time, the cats in a room down the hallway meowed loudly, and the farm animals bayed, neighed, and bleated. Not in a crescendo, one after the other, but all at once, at the top of their lungs—the instant Diamond died.

I had seen pets get agitated, pacing nervously, just before a house companion died. I'd witnessed them totally ignoring the deceased immediately after, as if they knew the life force was gone. However, I'd never before heard a cacophony like this. The animals kept up the ruckus for, maybe, thirty seconds or so. Then, just as suddenly, all was quiet at the farm. No creature made a sound.

With my stethoscope I listened to Diamond's chest. No heartbeat. I shook Mr.'s hand and gave him my heartfelt sympathy on the loss of his pet. A moment later, Mrs. entered the room, and I gave her my condolences. She put her arms around me and thanked me for coming. I replied, "And thank you for letting me help you with this difficult time." Mr. said he would bury Diamond on the property. They both thanked me again. Marsha and I left.

We rode all the way out the driveway without saying a word. Once on paved road, I asked her, "What happened? What did you hear?" I wondered if I imagined the howls. *Did I really hear what I thought I heard?*

"It was amazing. I was looking toward the house. Suddenly all the animals started making loud noises."

"So you heard it, too? It sounded like, not just the dogs and cats, but the horses, sheep, and their pig all wailed at the same time. Right?"

"Even the rooster crowed, as if it were time to get up in the morning."

"Strange," I mused.

"But that is not the strangest part. The strangest part," she continued, "was the glow of white light that lit up the roof just at the time the animals started to howl."

"What do you mean?"

"I don't know how to describe it. But there suddenly appeared a whitish glow in the air around the roof just above the living room. It flared up, like a flash, the animals started howling, and then the light vanished. Poof!"

"There was a noise when the light went away?"

"No, it just vanished suddenly," she added in a nervous laugh "Not a 'poof' sound. Just 'poof' it was gone."

"Did anything else happen that might have startled the animals at that moment?"

"No. No noise. No thunder. No nothing."

All the way home I pondered this mystery that surrounded Diamond's passing. It was not a coincidence. A memory of a similar incident, involving a light at the time of death, came back to me.

As best I recall it, a doctor friend of mine shared with me an incident that happened at his son's death. I think he was hoping I might have an explanation. He was agnostic. Yet, he witnessed a phenomenon that went against the notions he held that there is no passage to an afterlife, only blackness, nothingness.

His adult son, a competitive bike racer, was on a training ride early one Sunday morning through a city park. According to witnesses, a pickup truck going in the opposite direction of his son swerved deliberately into the bike path and hit his son head-on. A hit-and-run.

My friend was in a waiting area outside the emergency trauma room (ETR) of a hospital. The medical staff was frantically working to save his son's life. He told me that as he stared out the window, a bright but cloudy day, he saw a sudden flash of a blue light coming from the direction of the outside wall of the ETR. The light rapidly ascended in a flare into the clouds above and disappeared.

He asked himself, "What just happened?" Turning back to the room, he glanced at the clock on the wall. It read, *11:43:17 a.m.* He sat down and picked up one of the outdated waiting room magazines.

A few minutes later a doctor came into the room and approached him, "I'm so sorry. Your son passed away." Some tearful words were exchanged. Then my friend asked, "What time did he die?"

"Eleven forty-three."

17

Atlantis

January 5, 2007, 9:41 p.m.

Only now can I write of the event of two days, two nights and two hours ago.

Atlantis came home to die.

I was watching the Iowa caucuses' news on TV. Thunder and lightning, rain and high winds roared outside.

My wife, Marsha, was driving home. She squinted her eyes to see through the curtain of silver drops. As she was turning from our unpaved access road into the driveway, she spotted a black and white animal. "A skunk?" she wondered. It was a wet mop of a thing, climbing, struggling, over the embankment from the river, half in brown slurry. It fell in the mud unable to get up; rain pelting down. She slammed on her brakes, skidding a little as she was making the turn. She got out, lifted her raincoat up over her head, and peered at the object. Recognition flushed her face. She quickly scooped up the bedraggled creature and jumped back in the car, holding it in her lap on the drive up the pavement to our house.

When Marsha walked through the front door cradling the dripping mass of fur, it was clear that poor Atlantis, our eight-year-old male "tuxedo" cat, was in great distress. She explained to me how he had crawled up the embankment on the riverside and tried to cross the muddy road. But the struggle was too much. His energy gave out.

Atlantis had been missing for a week. He had shown the typical telltale gagging signs of trying to hack up a hairball—something he often did. I thought nothing of it until I noticed, as I was leaving for a house call, that he was heaving with nothing coming up. I made a mental note to examine him further when I returned. When I looked for him later, he was nowhere to be found.

I took Atlantis's limp body out of Marsha's arms and laid him down on the kitchen counter. He shuddered in spasms as if in pain. He was cold. I toweled the muddy water off his back and belly and placed him on a heating pad. He was dehydrated, so I gave him an injection of fluids. I gave him an injection for the pain as well. But, before any of the attempts at treatment could take effect and only a couple of minutes later, he jerked spasmodically, twisted his head back, his legs splayed out in front. He cried out, gasped once, and died.

Marsha then told me an incredible story.

Atlantis had been gone too long. We were worried. We pictured him sick, hiding out somewhere, alone, as cats are wont to do. She said that that very morning she had prayed to her mother to bring Atlantis home. Irene loved cats and disliked dogs. She often said she wanted to come back as a cat in her next life—to sit in someone's lap and be petted.

Irene and Atlantis were indelibly connected. You see, Atlantis was born in Irene's kitchen the day of her funeral.

I had arrived home only a half hour before Marsha. But Atlantis wasn't in the road when I drove in. Marsha's headlights spotted him climbing the embankment and onto the road. If he had come up just a little later or Marsha had driven up a little earlier, he would not have been seen. He would not have had the energy to make it up the long climb up our steep driveway to the house. We would have found his carcass on the road in the morning.

It was a miraculous sequence. My wife believes her mother helped Atlantis to Marsha's sight. Answering her prayer.

The veil between us and the other side is oh so thin.

After his death, not much more than fifteen minutes after bringing him inside the house, we held each other. Tears flowed. I felt bad that he had suffered so much pain before dying. We also cried because we were so thankful he died here at home, where he belonged, where we could touch him.

Atlantis lay dead, on his left side on the kitchen countertop where I had placed him. We spoke with blessings and thanks directly to his soul and to Irene's soul. At that precise moment Atlantis's right, upside, ear twitched. Unmistakable, as we both saw it. No other body part showed any postmortem movement. When he died I had listened with my stethoscope and confirmed that there was no breathing and no heartbeat. To us, the ear twitch was a physical sign from the other side. "We hear you."

So blessed, for the prayer that brought him home and for the physical evidence of communication from beyond.

I performed a necropsy (autopsy of an animal). There was a hole as big as my little finger in his esophagus and into his chest. Not an ulcer, but a penetration, a puncture. There was massive infection involving the lungs and heart. The chest cavity was filled with bloody pus. I did see a couple of pieces of brown remnants of vegetation. I couldn't find an intact foreign body, something that likely traveled through the esophagus and into the chest. My guess was the object was possibly a wood splinter or, more likely, a foxtail, a type of grass awn, well-known in California for its penetrating wounds. That examination revealed that I could not have saved him in his last moments. My sorrow and remorse is that I didn't attend to him in the early stages when the signs were those of a typical hairball.

May Atlantis rest in peace, a peace my haunting dreams may never have.

18

Cindy in Heaven

I always enjoyed going to Cindy Likens's house. When she opened the door it was like the sun bursting bright above the eastern horizon on a cloudless May morning. I would step inside her sanctuary of lanterns and flowers, always flowers on her fireplace mantel. Her tortoiseshell cat, Iliad, would run up and rub against my leg as if greeting an old friend rather than the one with the needle. This was followed by slow-moving old Homer, a mustached gray terrier, whose lick made up for the imbalance of his arthritis. He, too, forgave my pointed intrusions.

"Hello, Dr. MacVean. How about a cup of tea?" Cindy would usually ask. "And I have sugar cookies I just baked this morning," as if she were a grandmother rather than the twenty-eight-year-old cute blond who made me wish I was a couple of decades younger.

"Sure, I'll have a 'spot-o-tea' and a 'wee biscuit,' if you please," poking fun, as I always did, at her British heritage and my Scot ancestry and in anticipation of her inevitable "Oh, you" response while poking my belly as if I was the Pillsbury Doughboy.

Cindy was always positive. I felt good being around her since she let me know frequently how she would never have another vet treat her pets. "You're the best!" It is amazing to me how loyal some clients can be. She was a busy young lady, working full-time for the state, volunteering at Loaves and Fishes, the local feeding program for the homeless, going out with friends and on occasional dates.

My visits to her house were routine: annual physical exams and booster vaccinations. Occasionally there was nail trimming and anal sac emptying when Cindy would inform me that "It is time for 'you know what.' Homer is scooting along the rug and his nails are clicking when he walks across the linoleum. And Ilie is sharpening her claws on my bosom when she gives me her kneady love!"

She knew that a dog scooting its butt along the ground is not a sign of worms but usually indicates that its anal sacs are plugged up. There are two bladder-like sacs, one on each side of the rectum. These glands secrete a pasty fluid that has a distinct, and to us humans, a nasty smell whenever there is a bowel movement. It is a marker on the stool and the rectum that is unique to each individual, much like a fingerprint is to us. It's how one dog recognizes another by its poop or checks it out by sniffing its rear end. The glands release their contents normally when an animal defecates. The odorous extrusion no doubt lends some lubrication to the stool as it passes out the anus. When the glands get too full, as can happen if the opening gets plugged up, the dog tries to empty them by scooting along the ground. When they are unsuccessful, we veterinarians help by inserting a gloved finger into the rectum and teasing the anal sac material out. Thus, the "you know what" treatment.

But this day was not the happy routine. Even though I got a "cuppa" and a "biscuit," Cindy was not as bubbly and energetic as usual. She stared into space as if she wanted to ask something. She did.

"Where do pets go when they die?"

"What?" I said, hearing an unexpectedly serious question from her.

"I've been thinking. Do you know where pets go when they die?" Her eyes focused, locked on mine.

"Uh, well, I do get asked that question occasionally. But I'm never quite easy with my answer, Cindy. I don't know for sure. What brings that up?"

Ignoring my question, she continued, "But what do you think? What is your best guess? What do we know?"

"What we know is harder than what we think or believe."

She continued to press. "You've seen animals die. What do you think about it?"

"Gosh, I just know they are an energy body, a life force. A creature of God. Their essence, consciousness, must survive the death of their bodies. At least, that is what my heart tells me."

She smiled, nodding her head as if in agreement, and laughed out loud. "Oh, silly me, what do I know?" Then she turned my attention to getting the vaccinations, nail clipping, and anal sac emptying done. She said that she was expecting a phone call from her mother in a few minutes and that she would be on the phone for a "while." Hence her hurry to get on with it.

Mmm, this isn't like you. What's going on? I finished up with the pets, quickly downing the tea, exchanging small talk about the weather, and left, taking the tasty cookie with me.

On the next annual vet checkup visit, Cindy looked tired, and there were shadows under her eyes. Her lovely ivory skin was more pale than usual. Her voice was subdued. Her movements slow.

In response to my comment that she looked tired. She said, "Oh, yes, I feel very tired. All the time now." I told her she needed to see a doctor. She said she did, and she was having a lot of tests. I didn't probe further, and she didn't offer more. The curtains over her living room window were closed; her sanctuary dark. Wilted flowers drooped from the vase on the fireplace mantel.

But Homer with the wiggly tail and mustached grin did his part in lighting up the living room. I took care of him, and then turned my attention to Iliad, the rubbing machine at my feet. I commented that Iliad was thinning along the back and had lost some weight; the skin fold indicated some slight dehydration. Cindy confirmed my suspicion that Iliad was drinking a lot more water and that there were more clumps of urine in the litter box. Drinking more, but not enough to prevent the dehydration since so much fluid was going out in pee. I told Cindy that Iliad, being eight or nine years old, may have one of the problems that come with middle age and that we should do a blood test to check it out.

"No, Doctor, I can't do that. I have had so many tests myself and expenses that I've run out my checking account. I can't afford to pay for it now. She's still very active and eating like a horse."

"I'm sorry to hear about your expenses," I said, ignoring the issue concerning Iliad. Feeling like I knew her well enough to probe, I asked, "What is going on? What's wrong, Cindy?"

For a moment the sun came out. She smiled and said, "It's okay. I'm responding well to treatment. I will be just fine, so don't you worry about me."

"But . . ."

"We'll take care of Ilie's tests next time."

"Look, Cindy, as a minimum, let me give her an injection of fluids to at least temporarily rehydrate her." I had already completed the physical exam of Iliad, so I added, "Besides Iliad's weight loss, dehydration, excessive drinking, and big appetite, her heart rate is very fast. I think she might have hyperthyroidism, an overactive thyroid gland. That is a treatable condition, and . . ."

"If it's not much, let's treat her."

"No, Cindy, I need blood tests to rule that problem in or out. She might have some other problem, like kidney insufficiency or diabetes. It could be dangerous to treat without knowing for sure." I saw my chance here, so I asked, "Like you, Cindy, you are being treated, but your doctor knows what for. What are you being treated for?"

That sun again, even brighter, "I am doing well. I will be fine. Don't you worry about that." Then, as if to divert my attention, she said, "Go ahead and give her the fluids. I can afford that much, but the vaccinations will have to wait. Please."

Like the flowers on her mantel my feelings drooped, as all veterinarians do when economics gets in the way of the best care for an animal patient. But I felt even more sinking as I saw Cindy tire from standing and then sag down into her big armchair and not get up again during this visit. I administered fluids by injection under Iliad's skin. Cindy even had me fill out the check, which she slowly signed.

Three months later, Cindy's mother, Margaret, phoned. She said her daughter was sick and couldn't be at the house. She said, "I'm up from Los Angeles to help my daughter and can meet you there. Cindy's worried about Iliad's weight loss, and I'll take care of the costs."

We met at Cindy's now-dark home. Her mother opened the curtains wide to let the light in. No flowers on the mantel, just an empty vase.

Margaret greeted me with a handshake and a serious sad expression. "My daughter has cancer."

Cancer is such a general word. It evokes such feelings of horror.

All cancers are not equal. Some are curable, whether by surgery, chemo, radiation, or combinations thereof. I asked, "What kind?"

"Leukemia. She is undergoing chemotherapy injections. She seems to be heading to remission."

I asked a few more questions, technical, doctor curiosity. Never mind, cancer is cancer.

I went ahead withdrawing the blood and urine I needed for Iliad's tests. The lab tests did reveal that she had advanced indicators of loss of kidney function. The condition was close to or at the irreversible stage, kidney failure. This was no doubt secondary to the underlying cause, hyperthyroidism. Margaret elected the palliative pills for treatment of the thyroid condition rather than the curative surgery or radiation. Iliad would have to be on the pills for the rest of her life and would need fairly regular injections of fluids.

In order to see if the dosage needed adjusting, I needed a follow-up blood test a couple of weeks after Iliad was started on treatment. On my next visit Cindy was there.

Her head was bald, and she had a wool cap on. She was thin, and the ridges of her ribs rolled under her tight T-shirt. Her color looked somewhat better than the last time, a faint blush on her cheeks. "I'm not better," she announced. And with a strange half smile, she said, "I am terminal." Then she asked that question again.

"Where do pets go after they die? I think they will be in Heaven with me."

She persisted in her question. She said she really wanted my opinion. "What are your feelings?"

I told her I wasn't sure. I admitted that the question confused me. My feelings were, at that moment, of Cindy, not of the question. I grappled with rolling internal tides.

To avoid dealing directly with my turmoil I put on my academic hat and gave her a list of what some people thought—to Heaven, to the other side of the Rainbow Bridge, to our Heaven, to their kind's Heaven, to nowhere (just the end of life and no more consciousness), to be a spirit among nature, to reincarnate as another critter, to reincarnate as a relative (human) yet unborn, to float in the "ether," and on and on. And blah blah, the way I was beginning to feel.

Sweet, sad Cindy smiled, gently amused that I needed to give the laundry list. She then told me that she had no doubts. They would be in Heaven with her. She also added that they will run and play, bark and mew, knead and lick, and cuddle up in a chair with her. I smiled at the beauty of that. She continued, "And I don't want to wait. I am dying. I won't live the year out."

Then she asked me the bombshell. "Will you put them to sleep right after I die?"

My head spun, dizziness struck. I rocked on my heels and didn't hear her next words. I recovered my bearings and asked her, "What? Say again. I didn't hear."

She answered, "It is important we die close in time, so we can make the connection. I must not be far away from them when they die so they can join me."

Shaking my head and putting on an uncertain cloak of knowledge, I argued, "Distance and time don't necessarily mean anything in the Great Beyond, not what we think of here on earth."

Persisting, she said her meditations tell her that it does make a difference. "Iliad's and Homer's energies will be transformed into something else, not connected with me, if there is much time between mine and their deaths." With tears welling in her eyes, yet with firmness, she asked for my compassion to grant her wish.

She elaborated with a relevant tale. "My grandmother remained as a ghost on this earth waiting for her husband to join her. It was decades before Grandfather died. Grandmother was trapped in an in-between world, and so didn't join Grandfather in Heaven when he passed on. She remained stuck here, a ghost in the house she couldn't leave."

Cindy pleaded, "I can't bear being separated from my dear pets for eternity." She said she wanted the joy of being together with Iliad and Homer forever.

Then she added, "Please do this for me. And for them. Please."

I was stunned and torn. *Yes, Iliad is not keeping up with grooming and gets dehydrated despite drinking a lot more water and has a severe kidney disease in addition to the hyperthyroidism. Homer is*

slowing and has arthritis; but they are still relatively young, only middle-aged.

Cindy asked me again, tears streaming down her gaunt young cheeks.

My turmoil, like tulips in late spring, wilted. I agreed to help her. I wanted Cindy to die knowing her wishes would come true. I looked into the eyes of her two loved ones as they sat at the end of the carpet, looking at Cindy and her tears. I couldn't communicate with them, but what I did sense was the love they returned to Cindy. *They were her partners in this life.* She would need to think of how to time this impending event, and I felt I needed time for God's help not to rue this decision. We knew it could come at a moment's notice.

The day came. It was a few months later when Margaret called in the early morning and told me Cindy died a few hours ago and asked me to come over as fast as I could to euthanize the pets. Tears welled up and I nearly choked on my response of how I honored Cindy and could I call her back in a few minutes. "Yes."

It took me several minutes to compose myself. I had hoped it wouldn't come to this. My mind started to justify their deaths, as I had done on a few sleepless nights, reiterating my arguments. *They are middle-aged. Ilie has thyroid problems and kidney failure as well. Homer is arthritic.* And countering, *They don't kill people because they're middle-aged. . . . I'm middle-aged, for God's sake!* I shook it off as my heart flooded the scene and washed away my thoughts. I felt the reality of the promise I made to Cindy.

I phoned her mother back. She thanked me and told me that a family friend would be at the house to meet me. She said she couldn't be there. She couldn't bear to see the pets die. I had a flare of anger. *Does distance mean anything—you know they die, whether you're there or not.* Followed by an amending *You are not to judge another's heart.*

I met Sam at the now-barren house, no furniture, no rugs, no flower vase. He understood my dilemma, but he had agreed to play a part in this drama. He told me that he had arranged to have the pets cremated that very day. The ashes would be placed in the wooden casket with Cindy. *At least they're not placing cat and dog carcasses in the casket with Cindy* flashed through my mind. I asked where she would be buried.

Sam explained, "Not buried. She"—unable to say Cindy's name—"was not embalmed. Quick cremation; quick turnaround time. The ashes of all three will be placed together in a box. I've promised them I would spread their ashes on a field at a friend's property in the mountains. Margaret can't be there, but I will choose a bright summer day with skies so clear you can see forever—all the way to Heaven."

As time has passed, I've further explored the mysteries of faith and the afterlife. Cindy's beliefs and comments have stuck in my mind all these years. I think now I would be able to discuss the subject in more depth. Perhaps I could have imparted a different perspective—and maybe a different outcome for her pets. At least I am at peace in my dreams, picturing a heavenly warm day, wild grasses bowing from a gentle mountain breeze, a dog jumping nearby after a butterfly, a cat sleeping curled up in the lap of a radiant young woman sitting in a field of wildflowers.

19

Olympic Rings

For Carl Jung, the ring meant continuity and the human being.

In 1912, Pierre de Coubertin designed the Olympic symbol to represent the five continents involved in the Olympics. According to Coubertin, the ring colors with the white background stand for those colors which appeared on all the national flags of the world at that time. Coubertin thought the rings had deep significance for the union among men.

The rings are joined together, one ring intertwined in another—continuity. We strive through faith and love, even in the face of overwhelming odds.

The fighter enters the ring with determined intensity, focused willpower. To compete, to win, to stand on the winner's platform. Engage the battle. To its bitter end.

Oleg Olson was an Olympic kayaker—world class in slalom and sprint. He thrived on competition. He loved a girl. He adored a dog.

The latter is where I came into the ring.

I turned onto the dirt driveway. On a corner of the fence the bow half of a sawed-off kayak was stuck over a post. Oleg told me that was the marker for where to turn. The road wound a half mile through a grove of oak trees and over a wooden bridge that spanned a small creek. A creek that was dry now in the heat of midsummer.

As I approached the wood-frame house, it was apparent the structure had seen better days. Some of the roof shingles lay with upturned corners. The paint, once white but now gray, was peeling off the walls. Some of the porch and stair boards were loose or missing. A windowpane was cracked, the fissure partly covered with duct tape. A fading gray pickup was parked at the end of the drive on the north side of the house near the porch. Not much shade fell from the lone willow tree near the entrance to the house. Very little rain had fallen that summer. The willow branches were sagging, leaves yellowed, weeping.

I grabbed my medical kit, hopped out of my truck, and approached the porch. A short, thin man came out of the house to greet me. The screen door creaked as it slammed shut.

His grip was bony but strong as he folded his thin fingers and shook my hand. "Thank you for coming. I'm Oleg." His mouth curved in a half smile. Then the edges of his lips turned down. "Come in and meet my Champ."

Champ was a long-boned German shepherd. His haircoat was dull. He, no doubt, had been strong and robust in his younger days. He was now drawn, wasted muscles with thin sagging skin, and ribs standing out. His abdomen was swollen—a "cancer," Oleg said. Champ was Oleg's champion, fighting his illness for two years. A dog breed that loves to run, Champ tried his best to keep up sprinting along the river's edge with Oleg, even sometimes swimming alongside the kayak, right up until last month.

In a shaky voice, belying Oleg's strong brow and upright posture, he said, "My boy just lies there on the bed now. He can't get up anymore. He has always slept with me on this bed. He's my buddy, he . . . he . . . he's dying." Moisture glistened in the corner of his eyes.

I felt the welling of emotions, a dam about to burst.

"Damn it," he cried, flopping himself onto the fluffed-up covers beside Champ on the bed and pounding his fists into the abs of the mattress. A long silence.

I didn't want to talk, to interrupt the anguish. I felt awash in a flood of silence and awe. Even more so when he began to tell me his story.

Champ wasn't the only one who slept on the bed with him. In better days, his wife, Jill, Champ, and he gathered there at night, a bed of love.

Oleg spoke of Jill with reverence, though his voice caught on a word here and there as he told me of the bliss the two of them shared. They met at the Olympic Trials, introduced by a competitor of Oleg's. "Our eyes filled with stars," he explained of their first meeting. "There was no stopping our passion." *The Olympic flame*, I thought.

It was a happy and exciting marriage. Then Jill got sick. An ovarian cancer came on with indiscriminant rage. There was pain, a burst of the growth that spread throughout her abdomen. It reached an inoperable stage quickly. Her small frame dwindled.

"I fought with her, with the chemo," he said. "But I couldn't stop the suffering." He pounded the bedcovers once again.

I sat down on the edge of the bed, stroking Champ in silence while Oleg cried and damned God. What could I say? His misery was raw.

He sat up and lifted the edge of the bedspread to his eyes and wiped at his tears. "She died a year ago. We couldn't win," he sobbed.

My throat constricted, the words came out taut, "I . . . I'm so sorry." I reached over and squeezed his hunched shoulders.

"I've been helping, battling, along with Jill and Champ." *His loop of life.* I imagined I heard the words unspoken, "We are losing." *The loop of tragedy.*

I leaned over and palpated Champ's abdomen. I placed one hand under his belly and tapped on the opposite side, sending a pressure wave through his abdomen that I could feel with my hand on the underside. His abdomen was full of fluid typical of some cancers. My fingers felt a huge mass under the edge of the ribs where the liver is. With the stethoscope I listened hopelessly to his chest as it heaved in struggle for breath. *Metastatic in the lungs now.* "It is the right decision, Oleg, to let Champ go, releasing him from his pain."

"I know. I know. It is so hard. So goddamned hard." His voice increased in strength and loudness as he proclaimed, "What did they do to hurt anyone? Nothing. All we did was love each other."

Quietly, he eased his body over Champ and wrapped his arms around him.

I felt pain in my heart seeing him clasping Champ, as if to hold him back from where he had to go. I had to go on, do my job. I filled out the euthanasia form on my clipboard and handed it and a pen to Oleg to sign. He scrawled his signature slowly, with a drop of the pen on his last letter. I picked up the pen, then laid it and the clipboard aside.

Drawing up the dose of fatal chemicals into a large syringe— *Champ probably won't even feel the needle go in*—I asked Oleg to move over just enough for me to get in front and access a vein of a front leg. "Please keep hugging and stroking Champ. Talk to him. Hearing is the last sensation to go." I placed the tourniquet, inserted the needle, loosened the tourniquet, and pushed the plunger.

"I love you, my Champ. I love you. Go be with Jill now. With J-J-Jill." His voice trailed off, and deep sobs filled the room. And as Champ took his last breath, "Good-bye, Jill, m-m-my Jill, good-bye."

Pressing the stethoscope to Champ's chest, I listened. No heartbeat. "Champ is gone, Oleg." Pausing for breath, my throat felt tight. "You, you have my, my deepest sympathy." I put my arm around his shoulder. He cried, splayed over his dog. His final words broke over me like a rogue wave, sweeping me away in a sea of emotions.

"Jill died on this bed. Now Champ has died on this bed. Soon I will die here, too. They told me I have six months to live."

I couldn't speak as his words crushed the breath out of me. I simply picked up my bag, walked out to my truck, slammed the bag and clipboard onto the back seat, and climbed behind the wheel. I relieved Champ's suffering. Yet, I felt helpless. I couldn't relieve Oleg's pain.

The sorrow hurt, and tears were welling up in my eyelids. I could still hear sobs coming from inside the house as I drove away.

Stopping at the gate, I stared through blurred vision at the half kayak totem. *And the interlocking rings will be complete.*

20

The Passage Home

"Life is going forth; death is returning home."

—Lao-Tsu, *Daodejing*

"Dogs do not have many advantages over people, but one of them is extremely important: Euthanasia is not forbidden by law in their case; animals have the right to a merciful death."

—Milan Kundera, *The Unbearable Lightness of Being*

"What is death?" I am asked. I reply, "It is a passage. Home, I believe."

What I say—

"May I proceed?" After her affirmation, I let her know, "I'm injecting now." I explain to my client in some detail what will occur and how it is done. I show Mrs. Brown how to hold Vince, to comfort and quiet both. Her cat's namesake, her husband, Vincent, passed away last fall.

I crouch down to my knees, at patient level, apply the tourniquet, find the vein, and thread the fine needle in. I loosen the tourniquet and let her know, "The injection is painless, and Vince will relax and go to sleep almost immediately."

I tell her to talk to Vince if she feels comfortable doing that. "The last sensation to go is hearing. The last thing he will be conscious of is your voice." I pause, letting that idea settle in.

"May I proceed?" After her affirmation, I let her know, "I'm injecting now." Her voice and attention are quieting and soothing. I push the plunger of the syringe, and the pink liquid flows into her dear Vince's body.

What Vince feels—

A lead bucket placed over my head, resting heavy on my shoulders. Stifled, my senses leave me. The air is heavy. I can't see for the surrounding darkness, echoes of breathing. I am unaware of taking a breath. I am soothed by the sound of her voice, slowing, sending me to sleep.

What I feel—

My mind awakens. The shared pain of loss of a beloved. I must think, get out of the feeling or fall into the abyss of grief. I struggle with my vocal cords to say something profound or, at least, comforting. "I'm sorry for your loss," or "My sympathy to you," are all that I can manage.

I pat a shoulder. I shake hands with a firm grip, my other hand resting lightly on our clasped exchange. Tension between my eyebrows, my lips set to keep from trembling, underscoring the gravity of the moment. "It's all right, I understand your grief." Not knowing all she feels, just knowing grief. I take my medical bag to the car. I make room on the backseat for Vince.

Go on. Accomplish what must be accomplished. I bend over the now lifeless form, listening with my stethoscope to confirm the absence of heartbeat and breath. "My sympathy, Mrs. Brown" once more. Wrap the body in a towel, blanket, sheet, or sometimes plastic (so cold), lift up the form in my arms. Say good-bye and carry us both to my car. Caring to take Vince to where he will be given to cremation.

Relief of suffering. Driving on to my next client and patient. On autopilot, tunnel vision, having staved off the brunt of sensations.

Suddenly a blaring horn behind me reminds me to come back, notice the light has changed from red to green. A ringing in my ears.

. . . The last sensation to go is hearing . . .

Sometimes when I drive away from the house where I've just put a pet to sleep, I think "Where do the souls go?" They do seem to have souls—some life-force energy unexplained by a pumping heart and a thinking brain. Indeed, many fur-clad souls seem to vibrate at a higher level than some people I've known.

And what of life before death? The creatures we veterinarians deal with bring much love, comfort, and companionship to their people. Even an uplifting of spirits that can't be anything other than healthy.

Once I visited an elderly lady who was bedridden. The house was in a wealthy Sacramento neighborhood called the "Fab Forties." Mrs. Sophie Childress was dying of pancreatic cancer and was going downhill rapidly, given only a few days to live. Hospice care was assigned. Her hospice care nurse would come in the morning and leave in the evening. The lady's daughter would be there overnight and on weekends.

The nurse let me in the front door. Carol was a tall, slim woman in her thirties. Her dress was plain, but not medical garb. As she led me to the back bedroom she told me she was concerned that her patient was very worried about her cat.

"The worry, I feel, is bringing her downhill faster than the cancer. Her cat is so important to her. When Callie jumps up on the bed and settles in beside her, Sophie brightens up and her pain seems to subside. Pain, I know you know, increases blood pressure. The comfort and purring when she is petting Callie seems to help lower her blood pressure." Carol went on to explain that her patient often fell asleep after petting Callie for a while, her hand resting on Callie's back. I wouldn't be surprised if studies show a release of endorphins and serotonins moderate the perception of pain.

We reached the master bedroom, now an infirmary. Bare wood floors, two beds, both adjustable and on casters so they could be rolled to different locations in the room. On the wall, where Sophie could view it from where she lay in her bed, hung a reproduction of a painting of an old woman sitting in a big overstuffed chair with a cat in her lap, both looking at a bird at a feeder in a windowsill.

A scratching post with a lounging platform on top rested at a large bay window on my left. From where I stood, there was a clear view of the flower beds in the backyard. A hummingbird feeder suspended from a tree branch hung in view at the edge of the window.

In bed was a small thin woman with tissue-paper skin. Her skeletal arms rested on top of a colorful quilt that covered her body up to her chest. Her gray-white hair was cropped short, her cheeks gaunt, sunken in, as were her eyes. At the head of the bed was a fluids stand with a bag of saline and IV drip line that hung from it. Mrs. Childress was fast asleep. Callie, too, was napping right next to her side.

A middle-aged woman got up from a folding chair next to the bed. She was reading a notebook and quickly laid it on the small table next to the chair. A lamp behind the table lit the reading place. Unlike Carol or Sophie, she was broad-hipped and dressed in a white long-sleeved blouse and gray slacks.

"I'm Felicia, Sophie's daughter. I called you because Callie means so much to Mother, and I'm afraid Callie is sick. Callie has been vomiting of late." She told me she came to see her mom every day, "as soon as I can get my phone to stop ringing and my door closed." She ran her own business, dealing with legal drafts. "I sleep here, in that bed next to Mom. Carol leaves at night."

Upon questioning from me, Felicia added that her mom's cat appeared to be losing weight because "maybe she wasn't eating well." We placed Callie on a protruding shelf of the scratching post near the window. Callie could dig her claws into the carpet material covering the post. She was a spayed female long-haired calico, about six years old. The exam was routine. Everything checked out normal except for the soft, mushy feel of her stomach.

Felicia agreed to laboratory testing of blood and urine. The nurse was registered and was willing to do whatever was needed to help. "I have cats of my own," she said. Carol was quite capable at holding Callie while I obtained the blood and urine samples. I let them know the lab tests would be done overnight and that I would call them in the morning with the results.

"In the meantime, just in case my provisional diagnosis based on the exam and history is correct, we can treat for hairballs." I handed Felicia a tube of hairball paste and showed her how to administer it, giving the first dose myself. Callie licked some of the malty-smelling paste off my finger. I then opened Callie's mouth and smeared the remainder on the roof of her mouth. Callie licked and swallowed. "If she won't take it off your finger or doesn't let you press it in her mouth, you can smear it on her lips or on a paw. But rub it in good so she doesn't flick it off. Cats are so fastidious. Callie will lick her lips or paw clean."

Felicia offered to pour me a cup of coffee. "It's already made. I just had a cup. Or I can get you some water from the fridge."

I accepted the coffee, black. It was clear to me that Felicia wanted to talk a while, and my next appointment wasn't for another half hour and was in the same neighborhood.

Felicia told me how her mother smiled when she would see Callie on the scratch-post tower staring out the window. "Reading the newspaper," as her mom would say.

"Mom's husband was an engineer for the county. She lost him about twenty years ago. She loved doing all sorts of handicrafts, tole painting, and quilting." Pointing to the colorful spread I'd noticed on Sophie's bed, she said, "Mom made that quilt herself." Felicia added that her mom loved to play bridge with her lady friends.

I got a word or two in. "I play bridge also. Keeps the mind sharp." *Use it or lose it.*

I don't remember what other reminiscences she relayed, but soon it was time for me to go.

The next morning I called with the lab test results. "Blood and urine were all normal. So it is possibly a hairball after all. Just continue treatment as I explained. Once daily for seven consecutive days. Then three times weekly to prevent future hairballs from forming. And, please, call me if anything changes with Callie." Carol said she would pass the information on to Felicia.

A couple of weeks later I got a call from Carol. With a sorrowful tone of voice she informed me that Sophie passed away. She said Felicia woke in the morning and found that her mother was not breathing and immediately called for an ambulance. The paramedics confirmed death.

"Felicia was too upset to call you herself, but she wanted you to know that when she was cleaning the cat box last week she noticed that Callie had passed a stringy fur ball in the stool. She also wanted you to know that she would like you to continue seeing Callie. You know, exams, vaccinations, and so forth. And I just wanted to tell you that when I left Sophie the evening before she passed she was sound asleep with her hand over Callie."

Felicia did call a few weeks later. She told me she was convinced it was the love of her cat that kept her mother alive the precious extra weeks. "Oh, Callie is living with me now. She deserves the best. Before I could move the beds and prior to bringing her to my house, she would come and lie on Mom's bed every day, staring out the window, bird or no bird." A pause of thoughtfulness, then: "I wonder what she was thinking. Was she thinking of Mom and the times they, together, looked out at the trees and birds? Was she remembering the feel of Mom's lap? I wonder." A further pause. (I love how people share things with me.) "It's such a pleasure to me to watch Callie sit on her scratching post, looking out my window, reading the newspaper. I've even joined her. Sitting beside her I stare outside. I feel Mom's presence."

I continued to see Callie the next few years. Ultimately Callie didn't need my help in passage to the other side. As Felicia told me, "I found Callie curled up on top of the corner couch where I had placed my mom's quilt."

My aunt Clara was a tall woman with large bones and always carried a bit of "fluff" around her midsection. But not when I last visited her. She was eighty-four years old then, living alone in her home in Sacramento. She was always so very self-sufficient. Well, she wasn't really alone; she had her best friend, Sonny, sharing her house. Sonny was a twelve-year-old terrier/Labrador mix weighing around forty-five pounds. I would see him every so often to catch him up on vaccinations and renew the pain meds prescription for his arthritic hips.

I commented to Clara that she was getting thin. She said, "I feel nauseous most of the time and don't eat." Missing a meal was not something that occurred very often. She added, "It took me two weeks to get a doctor's appointment. I go tomorrow. My next-door neighbor'll drive me." The lack of appetite surprised me, but seeing a doctor was one of the last things she would do. That was my clue it must be serious. I found out later that she had neglected to reveal to me the detail of pain in her abdomen.

I also noticed Sonny was gaining weight. She laughed her usual loud guffaw, "Ha, ha, yes, he gets the food I don't eat." There was no point in telling my aunt not to feed her dog human food—she would just smile and say "Listen, Sonny," like maybe I was a dog too, "what do you know? You're just a vet. Har, har."

The next time I saw her my sister, Marjie, and I were standing by her deathbed at a care facility. Clara immensely opposed leaving her house. She wanted to die at home, "Where I belong!"

Marjie and I were her only living kin. The hospice care nurse told us she had inoperable stomach cancer that had reached the final stages and that she was being dosed heavily with pain medicine, at Clara's request.

I expected she would be out of it and not very coherent due to the drugs. But, no, she recognized her niece and nephew, greeting us with "What kind of trouble are you two up to now? Har, har."

We began talking to her and asked, "How are you doing?" Well, that wiped the laugh out of her mouth.

"I'm doing damn poorly, if you must know." She grabbed her stomach, which bulged under the sheet as if she had a football there. Grimacing like I've never seen her do even when she was being sarcastic about something, she added, "The pain. It hurts! It hurts! I tell the f***ing nurses to give me more morphine. They won't give me enough!"

She went on and on crying, describing the stabbing sensation in her belly with off-color language that often shaded her speech when she was drunk or in a mood. If the pain she felt from an automobile accident thirty years before (in which she broke nearly every bone in her body) was a 10 on a scale of 1–10, this pain was a 100!

The pain was even worse the next day we visited. The nurse said Clara was at maximum dose on the morphine. She also said Clara wanted her to give her more, to stop the pain, to end it all, and that Hell couldn't be any worse. Our aunt had led a hell-raising life and so believed there were many reasons she would end up in the fiery ovens rather than cavorting with angels in rainbows.

We couldn't converse with our aunt then as she was quite delirious and going in and out of consciousness. Nurse said there was one consistent request that came up many times the night before. Clara wanted to see Sonny one last time. It was against the care facility's policies to have animals on the premises.

Both Sis and I thought: "Nuts to policy. She is dying." Nurse winked and left the room.

Marjie and I had always had a strained relationship with our aunt due to her unseemly lifestyle and her sometimes abusive language toward us. So our affection was conditional—unlike Sonny's, which was the embodiment of unconditional love.

A neighborhood man, who had seen Sonny a number of times, had agreed to take the dog. He brought Sonny that night to Clara's bedside. The dog's tail fanned the air like a propeller and he whined, lunging so hard the man lost his grip on the leash. Sonny leaped up on the bed, crawled over Clara's stomach, and began licking all over her face, snuggling up as close as he could.

Clara sat straight up in her bed. Not waking up in pain, but in pure happiness, grinning from ear to ear at the sight of her beloved Sonny. The human-animal bond, the loving and hugging was as pure and as deep as anything I'd ever witnessed.

Eventually, all settled down. The morphine kicked in again; and Clara fell asleep in peace, an arm enfolding Sonny nestling beside her, next to her stomach.

The next morning Marjie and I were informed Clara had died.

She came to that bed in tears of pain, but she left in tears of joy. The joy that only Sonny could give her.

One of the sad things about life-and-death decisions involving animals is that often it is based on economics. "Can I afford treatment? Euthanasia is cheaper." This is cruelty to the pet's people. It is agonizing. The psychological pain often lingers for a long time.

You might say, "This must be the hardest part of your job." I assure you it is not. I am sad for you, you who must feel the loss and pain of departure. But, for me, I am grateful that you have asked me to help you with this difficult passage. And that the pet no longer will have to live a poor quality life, and can pass pain free into eternity. The way I look at it is that this final act is grace; it is relieving suffering. It is that relief of suffering I carry with me.

A few times a house call for euthanasia became a late-night vigil. It might begin after dinner hour, and not end until before breakfast.

One of those times was when I met Corrie. Her sweet cat, Sammie (Samantha), was dying.

The sun had set late that summer night, as it does in Daylight Savings Time. Corrie arrived home about the time I was parking at the curb. She introduced herself, not smiling, and told me to come on in. "She's in the back, in the utility room. I didn't want to remove her. I'm so glad I got back home in time, so you wouldn't have to wait for me. I dropped my daughter off at my husband's girlfriend's house. I didn't want her to see Sammie pass." Then, as if apologizing, she added, "I would want her to be here if she was old enough to understand. She's only eight. I did let her see a momma cat give birth to kittens once at the state fair. But I don't want her to . . ." Her voice trailed off.

I nodded. I'd heard that kind of comment only a little more often than I had people tell me they wanted their children to see it, to share in saying good-byes. I've conducted euthanasia with no one present, not even the person who called. And I've had audiences—including a gaggle of grandchildren, parents, and all ages in between standing witnessing passage of a beloved pet, some wailing aloud and others mourning in silence, and some others blowing a kiss, or not, and a few quickly leaving the room before the event was fully underway.

Sammie, a gray short-haired tabby, was lying on her side on a small fleece blanket on top of a cushion. Corrie sat down on the floor beside the cushion and began stroking her furry friend's head. Apparently this sixteen-year-old was dying of an intestinal lymphosarcoma, a sinister cancer. She didn't want to take her in to her regular vet's "cold steel table." "I want her to pass here at home in familiar comfort."

I kneeled down and looked Sammie over, petting in between Corrie's strokes. Thin, dehydrated. Eyes open, staring into space, unseeing. *Definitely ready to go.* She was out of it already. She didn't respond in any way to our touches. At this stage, she would not have cared nor noticed if she was on a cold steel table or on a soft warm blanket.

I wouldn't need to give a sedative to this patient. I could apply the tourniquet and give an intravenous injection straightaway. Corrie moved and laid down on the floor, face next to Sammie, and talked to her in a low, loving tone as I prepared the syringe. I administered the injection and listened to her heart. Breathing and heartbeat stopped. I reached over and patted Corrie's shoulder. "I'm so sorry, Sammie is gone."

Corrie rolled slightly onto her side and patted the floor next to her, clearly suggesting I lie next to her and Sammie. I didn't have another appointment after that and had already eaten dinner. I put my supplies away into my medical bag and laid belly-down on the floor. Corrie continued talking soothingly to her cat. She told her what a good girl she had been. She told me of the times in Sammie's life, and of hers.

"Love at first sight when I saw her at the shelter. I had to bring her home. They told me she was about eight years old and was affectionate and liked children. I was nine months along with Sally. 'Can you hold her until after my baby is born? I'll pay whatever boarding fees there are.' They were so kind. Sally has known Sammie all her life."

Corrie proceeded to tell me all sorts of things about their life together; the baby fun, the terrible twos, and the pretty little girl in ballet tutu. She also told me of the sorrow of her difficult marriage. She shared that, during the whole dreadful time, Sammie was her comfort blanket. How relaxing it was after a stressful day at work to have Sammie purring on her lap. Anyway, that was the gist. I'm not sure why I stayed so long, yet I felt good being there. It wasn't just *her* heart that was comforted sharing her experiences. The linoleum floor didn't even feel cold or hard. It wasn't until around 2:00 a.m. that she quietly finished her stories. I stood, telling her it was time for me to leave, and she had to get up early for work. She gave me a cup of herb tea. We hugged good-byes. She told me she would call me when she got her next animal, and I could then meet Sally.

The shared sadness and compassion bonded our doctor-client relationship from then on. It wasn't long after Sammie's passing that Beanie the beagle was brought into the house.

Over the years after that Corrie and I became friends, and she referred many new clients to me. I would visit a few times a year, usually for routine vet visits to see Beanie and the two cats she subsequently acquired. Sometimes the visit was social, sharing a beer or glass of wine. I saw Sally grow up. She wasn't a bad teenager at all. I witnessed the trauma of Corrie's divorce. I commiserated, sharing some details of my own divorce. I saw her achieve the release of recovery and the pangs and joys of dating. Sometimes I met the guy, and she would ask me my opinion afterward. "What do you think? A keeper?"

One day I was invited to come over to see her and Sally and "the brood." Corrie announced she was moving back to Colorado, "God's country," to the town she grew up in. "To start a new life. Home, where my heart is." And with a gorgeous smile added, "Maybe I'll find me a good cowboy to sink my spurs into."

She thanked me for being there. My heart melted. We hugged on the porch, saying our good-byes. She started to turn to go inside, and I turned to head down the steps. Corrie quickly turned back to me, kissed me on the lips, then hurried inside, closing the door behind her.

As I drove away, I asked myself, "Where is this place in Colorado?"

One of my favorite pieces of writing is for you, the special person who has loved a pet—

The Rainbow Bridge

There is a bridge connecting Heaven and Earth.
It is called the Rainbow Bridge because of its many colors.
Just this side of the Rainbow Bridge there is a land of
meadows, hills and valleys with lush green grass.

When a beloved pet dies, the pet goes to this place.
There is always food and water and warm spring weather.
The old and frail animals are young again. Those who are
maimed are made whole again. They play all day
with each other.

There is only one thing missing. They are not with
their special person who loved them on Earth. So, each day
they run and play until the day comes when one suddenly
stops playing and looks up. The nose twitches. The ears are up.
The eyes are searching. And this one suddenly runs from the group.

You have been seen, and when you and your special friend meet,
you take him or her in your arms and embrace. Your face is kissed
again and again, and you look once more
into the eyes of your trusting pet.

Then you cross the Rainbow Bridge together,
never again to be separated.

—Anonymous

21

Bad Dog—Good Dog

Okay. I'm an eternal optimist. Pets are good. Pets and their people are all good. It's rainbows and kittens.

That reflects my attitude, but not always reality. I've run into my share of aggressive animals. Mr. Chow (chapter 5) was an example of a "bad" dog. But how did he get that way?

Some breeds of dogs were wonderfully friendly companions in the days of my childhood. Spot, the cocker spaniel. Penny, the standard poodle. Goldie, the golden retriever. Suzie, the Australian shepherd. All desirable family pets. And many others of those breeds still are nice these days. But irresponsible inbreeding or deliberate genetic crossings of mean dogs have resulted in a higher frequency of individuals who can't be trusted. I've had clients tell me they can't have the "purebred" around their grandchildren because he or she will bite them.

Some will argue that a dog's disposition has more to do with upbringing. How you raise your pet, rather than a congenital defect. Some lines of Staffordshire terriers have been bred and trained specifically for game fighting other dogs in the pit, hence the name pit bulls. Pit bulls were originally kept as nanny dogs for nurturing and protecting small children. But look at their reputation now. Over seven hundred cities in forty states in the United States will not allow you to have a "pit bull" because some have mutilated children, chewing the skin off their face among other atrocities. Yet, I have come across many of my clients' pit bulls that are sweethearts. Many of these clients tell me it is because they are raised with love and treated with kindness in their upbringing. "Treat them mean, and they will be mean."

I must admit that I, too, had prejudices against certain breeds. I took the approach to those breeds that the pet I was examining could suddenly turn on me aggressively. It was not to be trusted. Muzzle him. "NO muzzle!" some clients would say to me. "He's as gentle as can be. He's never bitten anyone before," as Ms. Lyle said about Mr. Chow. I've forgone muzzles sometimes with good results, but sometimes with near misses of sharp fangs.

One day I was filling in at a veterinary hospital that was short of staff at the time. Carrie, who manages SIAR (Sacramento Independent Animal Rescuers), was at the hospital that day. She entered the office where I was sitting at my desk and told me a patient that was in for neutering was a rescue dog and needed a good home and asked me if I would like to adopt him. She knew my wife and I had lost our English springer spaniel to cancer several months earlier. "And you like nice dogs."

I told her I wasn't sure if I was ready yet. "What's he like?"

She said his name was Atticus and was as friendly as could be. "He's a pit bull about one and a half years old. He was picked up in South Sacramento. The owners abandoned him chained to a stake in a front yard. He's in the back kennel recovering from being neutered this morning. He's in great shape and has had all his shots."

My immediate response was, "No way. A pit bull? Are you kidding me?" I didn't realize how strong my distrust of the breed was until I blurted that out.

"Oh, Doctor MacVean, you should meet him. He's a honey."

My teenage granddaughter, Brazyl, who was doing volunteer work at the hospital that day, came out from the kennel area and walked into the office. "Papa, you *have* to take Atticus. He would be such a good companion for you and Grammy. He is the sweetest dog. He wags his tail and licks my hand."

"Look, dear, don't always trust a wagging tail. They can lick the skin off your hand—until they rip your hand off." (Such exaggeration to make a point!)

"But, he . . ."

"No pit bull. Period!"

With that, she spun on her heel with a pouty lip appropriate to her age and headed to a back room.

I turned to my desk to eat the sandwich I brought for lunch.

After I'd finished eating, a couple of the staff came by. We spent the next ten minutes or so discussing the idea of me getting another dog. I was thinking that the time of mourning had been over eight months now, so maybe it was time for another dog. But I had a picture in my mind of the pit bull ravaging our two cats.

Carrie continued standing and said, "You should think about it. You could take him home for a two-week trial. He is a great dog. A real looker."

Right then, Brazyl marched into the room with a grin on her face. "I just got off the phone with Grammy. She said it's okay and to bring Atticus home."

Ha, sneaky girl. Going behind my back. Clever, getting in through the back door. Later I learned that Brazyl, Carrie, and the other staff deliberately waited until I had lunch to approach me further about my taking the dog. They knew that I sometimes get grumpy when I'm hungry.

I did indeed feel better with lunch in my belly and my blood sugar level back up to normal, but I still held on to a bit of intransigence.

"Look, we don't need a dog who you can't know when he's going to turn on us. And I doubt Muu and Phantom would like having to hide out all the time for fear of being chased by a mad dog. Besides, we don't know anything about this beast that was chained up and abandoned. He was abandoned for a reason, you know."

"Well, Grammy said to go put him in the truck and take him home."

Turning to Carrie, I said, "What do we know about this dog? Nothing, other than being chained up in a yard before you guys picked him up. Right?"

"I'll find out." Carrie and the others walked off down the hall.

"Brazyl, isn't there a kennel that needs cleaning?"

As she ambled off toward the kennels, I heard Brazyl mutter over her shoulder in my direction, "Okay, but Grammy says . . ."

With a shake of my head, I turned back to the computer to enter my notes regarding the last patient I'd seen. A few minutes later Carrie entered the room and gave me the phone number of the woman who rescued the dog from the front yard. Carrie left. Hesitating before picking up the phone to call, I thought, *I hope she's not home, so I don't have to deal with it.* I picked up the receiver and dialed. *If I put it off long enough, maybe . . .*

"Hello." *Darn, no luck.*

"Hello, Mrs. Johnson, this is Dr. MacVean at Sylvan Corners Pet Hospital. I'm calling about Atticus."

"Oh. How is that darling baby doing? Is he okay?"

"Yeah, everything is fine. I just want some information about his history. What can you tell me?"

Boy, the floodgates gushed open. She told me how she saw him chained to a stake in the front yard of a house down a few doors from her house. "His owners, Mr. and Mrs. Garcia, left, moving all their stuff in the middle of the night a couple of days before I noticed he was still chained. My neighbors and I took turns feeding him and filling his water bowl. Surely they would come back and get him. He's such a beautiful dog. It's beyond me why they didn't take him with them."

Because he's a bad cur? "I haven't seen him yet, but I understand he is a pit bull. Can you tell me anything more?"

"Yes, a purebred bluenose. They kept him in great condition; and had him up to date on vaccinations, worming. They even paid for expensive ear cropping surgery to make him look, like, real macho; and they didn't want to neuter him for the same reason. Anyway, after three weeks they were still a no-show. We found out from their next door neighbor that they could no longer afford the mortgage so they abandoned their house. Just walked out, with no forwarding address, leaving Atticus only enough food and water for a day. Poor thing."

My heart twinged.

"They were intelligent people. Even thought to give him a distinguished name, you know, like, after the lawyer in that book *To Kill a Mockingbird.* They seemed to love him so much. I still can't understand it. But he did lose his job a couple months before, and they had a baby on the way."

It all happened during the most recent real estate crash. The housing market had not yet recovered, and struggling owners were dealing with short sales or bank foreclosures. "It sounds like the Garcias had overwhelming economic pressures. It doesn't mean they were bad people."

"None of the neighbors had anything negative to say about them. They always pretty much stuck to themselves, and they would take Atticus with them in their car to visit their friends. My husband agreed that we should take him in. He seemed like a nice dog, and it was three weeks that he had been chained in the yard. We felt sorry for him. I'm glad to know you guys are going to find a good home for Atticus."

"We will try our best." *We? What's this* we *business?* "Can you tell me anything more about him? What's his disposition?" And thinking about grandkids that come to visit and our cats, "Do you know if he is okay around children, other dogs, and cats? And how is he with people?"

"Oh, my God, we couldn't imagine a better angel. I must admit, like, we had those same concerns ourselves. We have two children, ages four and six, two cats, and four little dogs" (a dachshund, two Westies, and a toy poodle). "Atticus got along great with them all."

I'll bet he was grateful. He got a square meal and a warm place to hang out. My skepticism was hanging around, not letting go.

She added, "Atticus was our official door greeter when our friends and Mom and Dad would come over to the house. They all love him. We kept him for six weeks. Both my husband and I work. Between our jobs and day care for the kids, it was a difficult schedule for us."

"I'll bet." *You trusted enough to leave your pets alone with the pit bull?*

As if she heard my unspoken words, she said, "Atticus became our trusted guardian; but our doxy was the alpha of the pack." Then she added, "We asked everyone we knew if they would take him in. We were crowded in our tiny home, and our finances were stressed. Then a friend at work mentioned that dog rescue group."

"SIAR," I said.

"Yes. We were so happy when they said they would get him neutered and find a good home for him. He deserves the best!"

After assuring her Atticus would be well taken care of, I put the phone down wondering where his next home would be. *He's good with people, dogs, cats. Friendly. Well, guess I'd better go have a look. No harm in that.*

Harm? Where did that come from?

I walked down the hallway and opened the door to the back room. I thought he might still be recovering from surgery and be calm from lingering sedation. *His guard is less likely to be up.*

He was standing, with Brazyl sitting down on the floor next to him. She was petting him, and he was licking her face. *No, don't let him do that. You don't know him.*

He was handsome, I had to admit. His stocky posture was straight, the short haircoat a shiny charcoal brown, ears pointed and erect. There was a white spot on his nose with a blaze of white that streaked up between the eyes to his forehead.

He saw me. *Brace yourself. Here he comes.*

Atticus was the epitome of ebullience as he scurried across the tiles toward me, his whole body wiggling back and forth so that it seemed like the tail was wagging his body rather than the other way around. He looked up at me, panting and drooling with eagerness to greet me. I cautiously bent down and opened my arms. He lunged to me, licking my neck and settling deep into my grasp. It was over. I was hooked.

IV
Healing Arts

"Until one has loved an animal, a part of one's soul remains unawakened."

—Anatole France

"There are more things in heaven and earth, Horatio,
Than are dreamt of in your philosophy."

—William Shakespeare, *Hamlet*

22

Stork Angels

The connection, the magical bond, between people and their pets is astounding. I've had clients tell me, unapologetically, that they love their pet more than their spouse. But then, I also heard a couple of moms say they loved their pet more than their children. Their babies come out of their own bodies. Pets do not. However, pets do arrive via storks; what I call "Stork Angels." Of course, they have to be an angel in an *animal* form. What did you expect from me? Besides, they are born with wings; human angels have to earn them.

The unseen world is a landscape so vast we have difficulty conceiving or imaging it. It is so beyond what we can observe with our six senses. Even gifted psychics have scratched only the surface. We in the healing arts have seen miraculous changes, such as recoveries that can't be explained by "rational" science. Spontaneous regressions of cancers are not uncommon examples.

Most people I know have had an experience of advice or an event coming out of nowhere that glorifies their life in some way. "It just popped into my head." Or, "She just walked into my life." No, it was not an accident, albeit beneficial or seemingly a synchronicity (a meaningful coincidence). There are just too many recorded incidences in literature and, I dare guess, in the archives deep in the cosseted walls of the Vatican to deny that there are benevolent forces at work on the behalf of individuals. I include animals, not just people.

In chapter 16, there was that moment of spontaneous chorus of wailing among the animals nearby at the instant of death of one of their own. Did they recognize the passage of a soul? Did they witness something visual or have a collective experience of group grief or salute or recognition?

When a pet is put to sleep many clients want to have their other pet come and say good-bye. But my experience has been that virtually every time the other pet ignores the dead body. Do they sense that the life force has left? Do they know "Buster" is no longer here?

Yes, I believe an animal's life force is a "soul." Yes, it is a spiritual thing!

What do I mean by "Stork Angels bring an animal into your life to enrich or even save your soul or the creature's soul?"

So, Stork Angels at work. What popped into your head that whispered you should take in this abandoned dog? And it turned out to be a win-win situation where you got unconditional love and your pet got not only shelter and food but the love and comfort that it needed? Turn it around. What brought this kind soul to pick me up and take me home and give me a square meal and a warm cozy place to curl up? Answer that, dear reader.

My alignment with Atticus (chapter 21) is an example in my view of Stork Angels at work.

Yes, there would be many "rational" explanations. Many related to the aligning of coincidence and social needs. Many related to personal religious beliefs.

Coincidence? Really? The event that connected you and your pet turned out to be meaningful even beyond what you first imagined. Synchronicity is a blessing. Remember, it was meaningful to the animal also! Who gave it meaning? Your internal needs? The animal's internal needs? Some unknown Gestalt? God?

Some decision was made based on feelings, facts, or the flow of time. A decision that the moment to bless is now! From an unseen force? Why not the metaphor I call a *Stork Angel*? Rejoice in the angel of delivery. Delivery of newborn experience—you to precious love, and your new pet to precious life. Not to mention worthiness and value. Not to mention mental and physical health to you both.

Prayer has an effect on healing. The scientific evidence is sparse, but it is there. Larry Dossey, M.D., in his book *Healing Words: The Power of Prayer and the Practice of Medicine* and in his later books, reviewed the published evidence and gave many anecdotal examples as well. Those studies were centered on people. Who wants to see a major study on unseen forces healing animals? Plenty. But who would undertake it, and who would fund it?

For now, we are left with some scientific evidence and lots of anecdotal accounts. And beliefs, even faith.

In one area of Malaysia, on the island of Borneo, some aborigines believe in certain birds as conveyors of spirit healing. The stork is one of them, I was told. In my years of working in the jungles of Peninsular Malaysia I encountered a few times when shamans (indigenous healers) worked the magic of their prayers in spirit healing. In one case I witnessed, a Semang chieftain's son was very fond of a particular cat that lived with him in the village. The prayer was simple, but lengthy. It included the three items I think are essential to every prayer: intent, empathy, and gratitude.

Intent: the medicine man gave incantations to heal the feline patient of a severe catarrh (a mucus congestion that blocked the throat as well as the nose) and catatonia (stupor) that looked so bad to me that a veterinarian might well recommend euthanasia. **Empathy** (as expressed in transfer of energy and emotional attachment to the outcome): the shaman's tools of bird feathers, bones, and other objects not identifiable to me were waved about with great vigor, and the name of the chieftain and son were attached to the prayer almost like a statement that the healing was taking place at that very moment. **Gratitude**: words of thankfulness for healing were enthusiastically spoken (present and past tense), and objects were offered to the spirit that was called forth to heal the spirit in the cat. I visited the village the next morning and found the chieftain smiling and his son playing with a very animated cat that showed neither signs of respiratory distress nor any mucus discharge.

Intent initiates a prayer. Intent awakens the energy that heals and focuses attention in your and your pet's direction. If you don't ask, you don't receive. Consider what is the desired outcome. What is in your best interests? What is in your pet's best interests? The more specific you can make the intention, the more powerful the message. For example, "I ask for healing for my dog, Sparky. Heal Sparky of his affliction (name it). Make Sparky comfortable." Some people add "Whatever helps us and our relationship, but most of all whatever helps Sparky."

Empathy the way I mean it is a sincere connection of energetic attachment to the outcome. You've probably seen the Carl's Jr. ads urging "Eat like you mean it!" Well, say the prayer like you mean it. Feel the emotion attached to it; stream that energy toward the subject (animal, person, event, time flow, or object). And be sincere. If possible, to give it cosmic power, say it with a tone as if the healing is already a fact.

An "attitude of gratitude" is an essential element to successful prayer. Give thanks that the healing is happening. Often all that need be said is "Thank you." Be grateful that healing is right there in exactly the form that is best for all concerned. Many really good prayers have, so to speak, "fallen on deaf ears" due to the lack of gratitude. Think of how much more willing you are to help someone when they ask for it and they express appreciation for your help. Why would a "God" care about gratefulness, you might ask? Trust me, the Spirit cares.

It is my view that it doesn't matter whether you envision God, Great Spirit, or whomever or whatever energy that you believe provides the healing. It doesn't matter what spiritual persuasion you come from or whether you are spiritual at all. The source of healing is listening. Your intention, your empathic sincerity, your gratitude all matter.

Is prayer a panacea? No, but is there any harm in adding a prayer to our armament of therapeutic agents? I throw in a silent prayer pill; it costs nothing. Pharmaceuticals, surgeries, manipulations are all well and good, but throw in a tincture of prayer for good measure. What the heck, throw in a suffusion of prayer! It can be silent, with no need to be orated, to be effective in healing. Try it; you might like it.

Veterinarian Allen Shoen eloquently writes of the effects of love on healing in his book *Kindred Spirits*. Pets pick up our emotions, what it is we are feeling when our pet is sick. When exposed to negative emotions they might be feeling at the least confused and at the worst the same emotions that we are. It is a rough time for us all when our pet is sick or dying. But, as best you can, rather than expose your pet to your sorrow, misery, and worry, show your love. Love is the power emotion.

23

What's Wrong, Doc?

My first conversation with a client is usually phone contact. Early in the conversation the client tells me the signs of illness and why the client wants me to come out to the house. "She's drinking an awful lot of water, and she won't eat a thing. What's wrong with her, Doc?" Having heard this expectation that I must be a diagnostic genius and can tell just by hearing a description over the phone, I calmly respond, "I'll need to see her. It could be a number of possibilities," *already going through a differential of alternative explanations in my head.* "I have an opening at one p.m. or four p.m., depending on where you are located. Where are you?" Sometimes the answer has been, "At home." And so it goes.

More frequently than I want to count, I'm asked the "What's wrong" question as I'm beginning my physical exam and have been told only "He ain't doin' right." Veterinarians even have a code for that diagnosis—ADR.

One of the pleasures for me is unraveling the diagnosis, of solving the mystery of "cause." Sometimes we never find the basic underlying cause, only the immediate clinical condition. The latter may solve the puzzle of naming the problem and even lead to successful treatment, of signs if nothing else. Sometimes ("most of the time" according to some doctors) the condition will resolve on its own if you give it enough time. I've had occasions (such as seeing a lame dog) where I've laid hands on my patient, said a silent prayer, and performed an ordinary examination, and the patient suddenly is symptom free (the dog is running about the house as if nothing had ever been wrong). We veterinarians and doctors in other medical fields sometimes wonder if we've really done anything at all.

I've had clients ask, "When do you stop practicing and actually perform?" I usually see a tongue in cheek, but a few have asked that question seriously.

Caretakers always want us to *do* something. It's a pressure to treat, even if we don't yet know specifically what we are treating. Many veterinarians today practice "data-based" medicine, which is a good thing. It's always been practiced to varying degrees, but it has a name, "data-based," that is currently in vogue. What is meant by that is performing diagnostic tests to derive as much information (data) as possible before deciding on a diagnosis or course of action. Data obtained by testing blood and urine, X-rays, ultrasound, and all the other magical gadgets modern technology provides.

It is a wonderful thing to have all the information you can gather so you can narrow down the diagnosis from a differential list of possibilities. Most veterinarians will go ahead and treat signs before all the answers are in. We try to give at least some treatment, and at the same time adhere to the credo "do not harm."

I admire the "barefoot" doctors of Third World countries for doing as good a job as they do, even though they don't have access to sophisticated serum chemistry or X-ray machines. Many Third World doctors are skilled at diagnosing without machines, a challenge I have appreciated in my house-call practice.

I'm not suggesting avoiding diagnostic testing. I'm only saying much good medicine can be done using careful observation with the birth tools—eyes, ears, nose, hands, and heart—and asking a lot of questions regarding the pet's history. Sometimes when tests are foregone, the doctor must reach into him or herself and the patient. This experience, which I call "connection," is like a mental (add heart) scanner. And it happens in an instant. There is a sudden knowing. "A bird on my shoulder just told me," I might say.

Clients often forget to mention an important detail of the living conditions of their pet, and sometimes we don't ask the right questions. An advantage in a house-call situation is that I can see, hear, smell, and feel what is going on in the patient's environment, which can be of tremendous benefit in diagnosis. For example, I was asked to see a parakeet that was droopy ("ADR"), a nondescript condition of a lot of avian patients when first noticed to be sick. Chest auscultation revealed raspy lung sounds and congestion. It was when I noticed on a table near the bird's cage an ashtray with cigarette butts in it that I got a clue to what was going on. My client did not mention that she was a heavy smoker and that her smoking chair was right next to her bird's cage. But the evidence was in plain sight. Everything turned around; the bird was back to normal within a week of my client doing her smoking in a distant room or outside in the backyard.

Necessity is the mother of invention. This challenge happens quite a lot in the type of house-call practice I have. I work out of my vehicle and see patients in their home (or on occasion in "the back forty!"). I do not have an X-ray or ultrasound machine with me. I do have a cooler containing my pharmacy. Some house-call veterinarians have a van that is specially equipped with holding cages, diagnostic tools (X-ray, chemistry analyzer etc.), and surgery suite with anesthesia—a traveling hospital.

I feel I was lucky when I first began my house-call practice because I got turned down for a loan to buy one of those vans. Why lucky? Lower overhead and expenses for one, which I can pass on to my client. In addition, as I later came to appreciate, I was able to hone my observation and history-taking skills to a higher level than if I had those diagnostic tools "on board." At least, that is what I tell myself.

I could treat based on my temporary diagnosis. Some clients don't want to go further, or, I should say, don't want to spend any more money. They would say, "If 'Georgie' is not better in a couple of days, I'll call you 'n maybe treat with something else." Others wanted tests done, so I would take the lab specimens I needed and have the commercial laboratory courier pick up the specimens for overnight testing. The lab would fax or email the results to me, and I would call my client with the results the next morning. If the lab reports were contrary to my presumption, I could then modify treatment as needed.

In cases when my patient was sick to the point where a definitive diagnosis and treatment was needed right away, I didn't hesitate to refer the pet to a hospital where emergency aid could be obtained. One time, a client, John, who was handicapped and did not own a vehicle, had a dog, Chap, that I determined needed immediate hospitalization. Outspoken and cranky, John was on bad terms with his neighbors, had no relatives nearby, and a taxi couldn't get to the house fast enough. So I ended up chauffeuring them both to an emergency clinic in my car. Chap responded to treatment well, and both John and Chap got a taxi back home.

In cases where nonurgent surgery was needed, I could offer an option: referral to another veterinarian (a house-call vet with a van equipped for onboard surgery, or a hospital). Or, I would meet them at an agreed-upon time at a hospital where I had surgery privileges. Camaraderie is alive and well among veterinarians. I am very grateful to those veterinarians who allowed me to use their facilities. In the latter cases, I was charged a fee for nursing help and anesthesia at a discounted rate or was not charged at all, as professional courtesy. Billing clients was up to me.

Clients get to see what goes on during exams and treatments by a house-call veterinarian. Most of the time clients appreciate that. Nothing is secret. Sometimes it's not a good thing. There's always the risk of something going awry under view of a doting caretaker. An example of the latter is having to stab several times to hit an elusive vein for a blood sample or occasionally having to stick more than one vein in order to get an adequate sample. It can be quite embarrassing. When difficulties or mishaps occur in a back room of a hospital, no problem, the client is unaware of it. When these awkward events happen on a house call, a mystery in the minds of my clients is solved. They say, "So that's what goes on in the back room."

I would like it if my patients would talk to me, as if communicating with Dr. Dolittle. One thing I envy that physicians are privileged to is that their patients can tell them their symptoms (subjective experiences) and where it hurts. Instead, a vet must rely on signs (objective observations) and, often, the intuition of experience. Neonatal physicians and pediatricians experience practice difficulties associated with lack of communication from their patients and in giving injections into tiny veins, etc., just as veterinarians do. I feel some comfort in that I am not alone.

Considering the difficulties of patients who can't tell me what is wrong and the sometimes bizarre happenings on a house call, it is not surprising that I have been asked on occasion, "Why do you still do this?"

The answer to that question is easy. "Because I enjoy it." I may come home from house calls at the end of a long day bone-tired, but I feel psychologically energized with that feeling that can't be beat. I know I have helped pets and the people who care for them.

To paraphrase Forest Witcraft, a hundred years from now, it will not matter the sort of house I lived in, what my bank account was, or the car I drove, but the world may be different because I was important in the life of animals and the people who cared for them.

Acknowledgments

Many thanks to all the veterinarians who helped me in my transition from academia to private practice. I especially thank Drs. Jay Griffiths and Narciso Lapuz for their advice and for sharing clinical and surgical secrets with me. They further allowed me the use of their facilities to sharpen my surgical skills. It was Dr. Lapuz who suggested that I use my wildlife veterinary experience as a house-call veterinarian. I've never regretted this career change, which has been so rewarding in the people and pets I've met.

I am forever grateful to my clients who gave me the privilege of entering their homes and providing me with the opportunity to help them and their beloved pets.

Much appreciation goes out to the members of the El Dorado Writers' Guild for constructive critiques and loving support that have helped strengthen this book. Encouragement from agents Jennifer Tran and Brenda Knight were like warm blankets. Special thanks go to Barbara Fleming and to Marsha Jacobson for their editing suggestions and confidence in the formation of the book. Thank you, Barbara, for your enthusiasm in getting me started on this project.

Many thanks to Nicole Frail, Chamois Holschuh, Chris Schultz, and Emily Shields of Skyhorse Publishing for their help in polishing this final product.